Student Bodies

CONVERSATIONS IN MEDICINE AND SOCIETY

The Conversations in Medicine and Society series publishes innovative, accessible, and provocative books on a range of topics related to health, society, culture, and policy in modern America (1900 to the present). Current and upcoming titles focus on the historical, social, and cultural dimensions of health and sickness, public policy, medical professionalization, and subjective experiences of illness.

Series Editors
Howard Markel and Alexandra Minna Stern,
University of Michigan

Formative Years: Children's Health in the United States, 1800–2000
edited by Alexandra Minna Stern and Howard Markel

The DNA Mystique: The Gene as Cultural Icon
by Dorothy Nelkin and M. Susan Lindee

Universal Coverage: The Elusive Quest for National Health Insurance
by Rick Mayes

The Midnight Meal and Other Essays About Doctors, Patients, and Medicine
by Jerome Lowenstein

Deadly Dust: Silicosis and the On-Going Struggle to Protect Workers' Health
by David Rosner and Gerald Markowitz

Inside/Outside: A Physician's Journey with Breast Cancer
by Janet R. Gilsdorf

White Coat, Clenched Fist: The Political Education of an American Physician
by Fitzhugh Mullan

Ordinary Life: A Memoir of Illness
by Kathlyn Conway

Student Bodies: The Influence of Student Health Services in American Society and Medicine
by Heather Munro Prescott

Student Bodies

The Influence of

STUDENT HEALTH SERVICES *in*

AMERICAN SOCIETY *&* MEDICINE

Heather Munro Prescott

THE UNIVERSITY OF MICHIGAN PRESS • ANN ARBOR

Published in the United States of America by
The University of Michigan Press
Manufactured in the United States of America
♾ Printed on acid-free paper

2010 2009 2008 2007 4 3 2 1

A CIP catalog record for this book is available from the British Library.

Library of Congress Cataloging-in-Publication Data

Prescott, Heather Munro.
Student bodies : the influence of student health services in American society and medicine / Heather Munro Prescott.
p. ; cm. — (Conversations in medicine and society)
Includes bibliographical references and index.
ISBN-13: 978-0-472-11608-9 (cloth : alk. paper)
ISBN-10: 0-472-11608-8 (cloth : alk. paper)
1. College students—Health and hygiene—United States—History. 2. College students—Medical care—United States—History. 3. Universities and colleges—United States—Sanitary affairs—History. I. Title. II. Series.
[DNLM: 1. Student Health Services—history—United States. 2. History, 19th Century—United States. 3. History, 20th Century—United States. WA 11 AA1 P931s 2007]

LB3497.3.P74 2007
378.1'971—dc22 2007020851

Foreword

ALEXANDRA MINNA STERN
& HOWARD MARKEL

Today, almost any college student suffering from seasonal allergies, in need of a flu shot, or interested in contraception takes access to the university health service for granted. Little does he or she know that this now integral part of the university system has a long and fascinating history that stands at the intersection of medicine, education, and adolescent health.

Luckily for us, Heather Munro Prescott explores this important topic in *Student Bodies: The Influence of Student Health Services in American Society and Medicine.* The result of extensive research in university archives throughout the country and informed by the author's broad expertise in the history of child and adolescent health, this book traces the evolution of university and college health services from the mid–nineteenth century to the present. As Prescott demonstrates, this is a story of how medical advancements and priorities affected young Americans as well as a tale of "bringing outsiders in"—of the increasing diversification of student bodies in terms of gender, race, ethnicity, and other forms of social identity.

As Prescott insightfully shows, the concerns and capacities of university health services were shaped by the context and era in which they arose. For example, at the turn of the twentieth century, apprehension over the university admittance of the "weaker sex" was often expressed as admonitions about women's supposedly frailer physical constitution and the potential damage that increased brain activity might have on the female reproductive system. Such gender anxiety in turn affected men, who were expected both to acquire the manly skills of rational thinking and athletic vigor and to avoid the menace of "unnatural" homosocial intimacy. This was the case at white- as well as black-serving universities, such as Tuskegee and Howard, where faculty and administrators were particularly concerned with properly educating young African American men to "uplift the race."

Later, during the tumultuous 1960s and 1970s, universities frequently became the epicenters of student protest. Clamors for the transformation of many aspects of student life and campus administration, including health services, were heard from Cambridge to Berkeley. Many student activists were incensed by the perceived medical paternalism of campus doctors, and various constituencies, including ethnic minorities, the disabled, and gays and lesbians, demanded representation on university health boards as well as in national groups such as the American College Health Association. This process only intensified with the appearance of AIDS in the 1980s, as many students insisted on HIV testing and "safe sex" education, which eventually became a routine part of life for most young Americans in college.

Anyone who has attended college or university will recognize many of the book's overarching themes. Indeed, *Student Bodies* aptly illustrates the adage that the more things change, the more they remain they same. College students long have been understood as a vulnerable group making the delicate transition into adulthood and autonomy. It is striking that more than 150 years ago, the faculty at Amherst College warned parents of the "dangers" particular to "College life," citing drunkenness, smoking, sexual improprieties, and gambling, among many others, as potential problems. Fast-forward to today, when parents and faculty alike share many of the same concerns about the deleterious impact of binge drinking, unhealthy eating, and drug abuse on college students.

Just as *Student Bodies* documents how universities and key organizations such as the American College Health Association and the American Social Hygiene Association helped to create the specialized field of college health and mechanisms for prepaid health coverage, the book also emphasizes the critical role of students as historical actors. This message could not be more relevant today, when the percentage of high school graduates enrolled in college or universities is at a historic high of nearly 70 percent. If we care about the generations who will lead this country into the future, it behooves us to care about access to and the quality of health services at American college and universities. *Student Bodies* illuminates how university health services developed over time to become what they are today; a wide set of stakeholders—students, faculty, administrators, doctors, nurses, educators, and lawmakers—will determine the future role of these services.

Acknowledgments

Numerous institutions and individuals have helped me during the decade I spent researching and writing this book. Generous support from the National Endowment for the Humanities (Grant no. FB 51467-05) and the National Library of Medicine (Grant no. R01 LM 8356-01), in conjunction with sabbatical leaves and Faculty Research Grants provided by Central Connecticut State University, funded the extensive travel to archives and time away from teaching necessary to bring this project to fruition. I am grateful to former Sponsored Programs director Dean Kleinert for helping me with these grant applications. I have also been fortunate to receive travel grants from the Bentley Historical Library at the University of Michigan; the Francis C. Wood Institute of the College of Physicians of Philadelphia; the Rockefeller Archive Center in North Tarrytown, New York; and the Sallie Bingham Center for Women's History at Duke University. The views contained in this book are my own and do not necessarily reflect those of these institutions or agencies.

Numerous archivists and librarians have helped with the research on this project. At Central Connecticut State University, I am especially indebted to the tireless efforts of Interlibrary Loan librarian Kimberly Farrington and her staff for their speed and efficiency in handling my voluminous requests. Radcliffe archivist Jane Knowles, reference head Ellen Shea, and other staff at the Arthur and Elizabeth Schlesinger Library on the History of Women in America have provided invaluable assistance throughout this project, beginning when I was an honorary visiting scholar at the library in 1998–99. My first foray into the history of college health was during my graduate studies at Cornell University, where archivists Gould Colman and Elaine Engst helped me piece together the story of 1903 typhoid epidemic. Other archivists and librarians who have assisted me extensively include Peter Nelson at Amherst College; David Kessler and Baiba Strads at the University of California, Berkeley's Bancroft Library; Karen Jania, Nancy Bartlett, Brian Williams, and William Wallach at the Bentley Historical Library at the University of Michigan, Ann Arbor; Laura Micham and Kelly Wooten at the Sallie Bingham Center at Duke University; manuscript curator Joellen ElBashir at Howard University's Moorland-Spingarn Research Center; Stephen Greenberg at the National Library of Medicine; Erwin Levold, Thomas Rosenbaum, and Darwin Stapleton at the Rockefeller Archive Center; Margaret Jessup, assistant curator of the Sophia Smith Collection at Smith College; Stanford University archivist Margaret Kimball; David J. Klaasen, Linnea Anderson, Dagmar Getz, Elizabeth Kaplan, and Karen Klinkenberg in the Anderson Library at the University of Minnesota; University of Pennsylvania archivist Nancy Miller; Diane Kaplan and Nancy Lyon at the Sterling Memorial Library at Yale University; and Toby Appel, Bumstead Librarian for Medical History, at the Yale Medical Historical Library.

Various college and university health care professionals have offered me insight and advice into the development of their field. I am especially grateful to Duke's retired health service director, William Christmas, for sharing the wealth of information on college health history he has collected over the years and giving me tips on the collections at American College Health Association headquarters in Linthicum, Maryland. I also thank Harvard University Health Services director David S. Rosenthal for helping me gain access to materials in the Harvard Archives. My colleagues in Central Connecticut State University's Student Health Service, Myra Rosenberg and Bosha Gordon, have also been supportive and shared insights into contemporary issues in student health.

Portions of chapters 3 and 5 appeared in the following publications and I am thankful to the publishers for permission to include portions of the material here: "Sending Their Sons into Danger: Cornell University and the Ithaca Typhoid Epidemic of 1903," *New York History* 78, no. 3 (1997): 273–308; "The 'Agrarian Myth' and Student Health at the University of Pennsylvania," *Transactions and Studies of the College of Physicians of Philadelphia*, ser. 5, no. 21 (1999): 87–117; "The White Plague Goes to College: Tuberculosis Prevention Programs in Colleges and Universities, 1920–1960," *Bulletin of the History of Medicine* 74, no. 4 (2000): 735–72.

For assistance in researching this book, I thank Cynthia Riccio, who served as history department graduate assistant during a critical stage of this project. I am also very thankful to the friends and colleagues who have read and commented on this work in progress, including Rima Apple, Nancy Bristow, Janet Golden, Wendy Kline, Susan Lederer, Richard Meckel, Danelle Moon, Ellen More, Elizabeth Toon, Sarah Tracy, and Elizabeth Watkins. I thank Kathleen Jones for sharing with me her unpublished work on college mental hygienists. Special thanks go to Margaret Humphreys and Alexandra Minna Stern for not only offering comments on my work but also allowing me to stay in their homes while conducting archival research.

My colleagues in the history department at Central Connecticut have provided invaluable encouragement, especially during the stressful years when I served as department chair. Briann Greenfield, Katherine Hermes, and Louise Williams were especially supportive. I am also grateful to friends from other departments who have offered insights from different disciplinary perspectives, especially professor of counseling Jane Fried, who commented extensively on the materials on college mental hygiene.

Finally, I thank my family for their love and encouragement. My parents, Dave and Sally Munro, worked at Dartmouth College and Mary Hitchcock Memorial Hospital, respectively, and were excited to learn more about the history of "Dick's House" and similar services for students around the country. My sisters, Hope Munro Smith and Sara Munro, have also been enthusiastic about the project and have given suggestions on how to make the book more readable to nonspecialists. Most of all, I thank my husband, Wayne, for enduring my frequent travels to archives as well as my emotional ups and downs as I finished the final manuscript. He reminds me not to take myself too seriously and to appreciate the wonders of life outside academia.

Contents

Introduction

In an 1845 circular to parents, Amherst College faculty warned of the numerous "dangers [that] attend College life." The circular described frequent cases of drunkenness, solicitation of prostitutes, gambling, smoking, and other habits "unfavorable to study and morality" among Amherst students. These accounts will probably be familiar to modern faculty, students, administrators, and parents. Stories about the health risks faced by modern college students regularly make headlines both in journals of higher education and in the popular press. College health professionals face continual pressure to do something about major health crises such as sexually transmitted diseases, depression, binge drinking, and epidemics of meningitis and other contagious diseases as well as to deal with more mundane yet more common issues such as managing chronic illness, preventing obesity, and encouraging regular exercise and healthy eating habits. These ongoing student health problems have led parents increasingly to demand that institutions of higher education take responsibility for the well-being of the student body. Baby boomer parents who once protested against parental rules on campus now suggest that colleges and universities return to a variation on their traditional role in loco parentis. College health professionals write of the frustrations of combating high-risk behaviors while respecting students' adult status and the need to promote independence and self-sufficiency.

When I reflect on my undergraduate experience at the University of Vermont in the early 1980s, I share some of this ambivalence about the best ways to protect student bodies while promoting personal autonomy and freedom of thought. I saw many of my classmates suffer alcohol problems exacerbated by the institution's reputation as a top "party school" in a state with a legal drinking age of eighteen. Like my classmates, though, I enjoyed the freedom and independence of college life. As a resident assistant, I was faced with the frustration of trying to control excessive drinking and obnoxious behavior without violating students' rights as adults. That same year, I took a seminar on the works of Michel Foucault, a scholar in residence during part of the fall 1983 semester. I was struck by some of the similarities between Foucault's ideas about the social construction of disciplinary institutions such as prisons, clinics, and asylums and the rules and regulations my supervisors in Residential Life expected me to enforce. I eventually wrote a seminar paper on the history of dormitories as institutions of social control. Ironically, Foucault's death from AIDS made tragically clear the limits of social constructivist interpretations of medical history. My experience as a client of the University Health and Counseling Services also demonstrated the shortcomings of Foucault's work, since it did not fully consider the perspectives of patients and their families.

Still, Foucault's ideas remained with me as I went on to graduate study at Cornell University. My graduate work in the social history of medicine and women's studies gave me a more nuanced view of the social construction of knowledge than that provided by Foucault. My courses illustrated the ways in which medical theory and practice both reflected and reinforced gender norms, racial stereotypes, and social hierarchies. Yet I also learned that clients were not passive victims of medical opinion and social control. Instead, patients and their families played an active role in the clinic and at the bedside, arguing with doctors, shopping around for care that suited their needs and pocketbooks, accepting and ignoring expert advice as they saw fit. My dissertation, later published as *"A Doctor of Their Own": The History of Adolescent Medicine*, examined the social, cultural, and scientific factors that shaped the emergence of this new subspecialty. I focused on how parents—and, more importantly, teenagers themselves—shaped the field of adolescent medicine.

Student Bodies extends this story into the young adult years, illustrating how college and university health programs evolved in conjunction with shifting standards of medical care and public health practices in the United States. College health is not a specialty in the classic sense, since there is no medical board specifically for that field. Nevertheless, there is a professional organization, the American College Health Association, which publishes the *Journal of American College Health*. Experts in this field make special knowledge claims for a particular class of patient based on their age and circumstances, a process that in some ways emulates the emergence of adolescent medicine as a subspecialty. Indeed, a number of college physicians today receive fellowships in adolescent medicine and/or attend meetings of the Society for Adolescent Medicine (SAM). The *Journal of Adolescent Health* frequently publishes articles on college student health issues. In 1995, SAM adopted a position statement declaring that adolescent medicine covered the ages between ten and twenty-five. The theme for SAM's 2005 annual meeting was the young adult/older adolescent. SAM advises parents about how to ensure that their children make healthy adjustments to college. Therefore, considerable overlap exists between the two fields, and college health can to some extent be seen as an extension of adolescent medicine into the college years. Some members of SAM have argued that the age of adolescence should be extended to cover the late twenties and early thirties to reflect the fact that the period of semidependency usually associated with adolescence has been extended because of longer periods of education, preparation for careers, and/or economic dependence on parents.

This book also examines the relationship between the development of college health as a field and the social construction of young adulthood as a life stage. I argue that college health programs did not emerge sui generis but rather were intertwined with the dramatic expansion of higher education in the late nineteenth and early twentieth centuries. Those who had formerly been excluded from elite antebellum colleges—women, blacks, recent immigrants—flocked to the new women's colleges and coeducational public and private universities created in the years following the Civil War. By the 1920s, growing numbers of parents and young people—especially those from racial and ethnic minorities—saw higher education as a means of upward social and economic mobility. Although elite colleges tended to reinforce the status quo by using entrance physical examinations to deny admission to those with "undesirable" physical and mental characteristics, public institutions and more progressive private ones used college hygiene programs to salvage and even rehabilitate unhealthy student bodies. Thus, expanding preventive health measures and clinical services became a way for institutions to deal with the new issues created by an increasingly diverse student population.

Most importantly, this book shows the central role students and their parents played in legitimizing the professional aspirations of college health experts. It explores the ways in which students shaped or even thwarted experts' attempts to regulate the student body. Gender role expectations strongly influenced the success or failure of students' strategies of resistance. The sexual double standard, combined with administrators' eagerness to retain men as clients, ensured that male students were less likely to face restrictions on their behavior than were female students.

To understand how health policies were implemented on the local level, this book draws on archival collections at Amherst College, Cornell University, Dartmouth College, Harvard University, Howard University, Radcliffe College, Smith College, Stanford University, the University of California at Berkeley, the University of Michigan, the University of Minnesota, the University of North Carolina at Chapel Hill, the University of Pennsylvania, and Yale University. I selected these institutions to provide regional and racial diversity as well as a mixture of public and private four-year institutions. More importantly, these institutions have the richest archival records on student health. To extend the story to a broader range of institutions, I have also relied on national surveys, published articles and books, data from funding agencies such as the Commonwealth Fund and the Rockefeller Foundation, and the records of the American College Health Association, which are split between Stanford University and the association's headquarters in Linthicum, Maryland.

Chapter 1 illustrates how gender norms and anxieties about female health shaped the higher education experience for women at both single-sex and coeducational institutions. It shows how the earliest college health programs emerged in response to ambivalent attitudes toward women's higher education in the late nineteenth century. Notions of women's traditional roles as mothers and the need to create an inexpensive and abundant teaching force to staff the nation's public schools promoted expanding educational opportunities for women. Yet this desire to "educate the race" via women conflicted with anxieties about "race suicide" of the white, native-born middle classes as it became apparent that female college graduates were less likely to marry and that those who did had fewer children than women who did not attend college. Members of the emerging black middle class shared these concerns that using educated women as a means of racial uplift would contribute to lower rates of marriage and childbirth among the black elite. They were also concerned that racial segregation and white prejudice made young black women more vulnerable to health problems. In some ways, those who supported collegiate-level study for women were quite progressive for their day in that they believed that women deserved the same education as could be had at elite men's colleges. However, they were also influenced by the work of physicians who warned of the dangers of higher education to women's health and took special pains to protect female student bodies by mandating regular habits regarding sleep, diet, and above all physical exercise. The dearth of reliable medical therapies at this time led many physicians to advocate a shift from curative medicine to hygienic improvements and state-sponsored preventive medicine measures, including mandatory physical education for schools and colleges. Teaching physical education and hygiene at women's colleges became a common career path for female physicians in the nineteenth and early twentieth centuries, a time when there were few other professional options for women with medical degrees.

Chapter 2 shows how concerns about race suicide shaped the development of health programs for men just as they did for women. Educators and medical experts claimed that excessive study caused nervous ailments and that white college men appeared to be smaller and less physically fit than men from racial and ethnic minorities. African American leaders also became concerned about the health of the elite young men who would go on to lead and strengthen the race as a whole. Men's colleges and coeducational universities in the period after the Civil War created physical education programs and athletic departments for male students as a way of ensuring that college men's bodies were as well developed as their minds. College officials also recognized that physical activity could be used as a way to divert male students away from "unwholesome" pursuits such as smoking, drinking, and illicit sexual activity. This desire to make college men manly yet moral was especially critical to administrators and health professionals at historically black institutions, who sought to overcome stereotypes about black male sexuality. College health officials had to modify their policies to suit student interests. Nowhere was this struggle between institutional control and student autonomy more apparent than in college athletics, which originated as informal contests organized by students and alumni. College physicians initially attempted to ban these activities, since the brutality of early contests resulted in high rates of injury and death. Yet student protests were so great that college health officials eventually had to recognize the limits of their efforts to combat the elitism of college athletics and promote exercise for all.

Chapter 3 examines the impact of sanitary science and bacteriology on college hygiene programs as well as conflicts between town and gown over attempts to protect student bodies from epidemic disease. It focuses on two case studies—the University of Pennsylvania and Cornell University—to illustrate the differences between urban and rural solutions to public health issues. Once again, notions of gender as well as race and ethnicity shaped how particular campuses responded to threats of epidemics and contagious disease. Warnings about the allegedly harmful affects of higher education on the health of young women led women's colleges and coeducational institutions alike to impose parietal rules that required women to live on campus, where their moral and physical well-being could be closely monitored. During most of the nineteenth century, officials were reluctant to assume the same responsibility for male students, largely because they believed that doing so was superfluous. After the Civil War, the average age of male students had increased to eighteen, and many administrators believed that men did not need the close supervision that had been imposed on the young boys who had previously attended college. By the early twentieth century, many parents found this situation increasingly intolerable, believing that their sons needed as much supervision as did their daughters. These efforts were constrained by fears that too many controls over male campus life would "feminize" men as well by as strong resistance from male undergraduates. These concerns about preserving gender role norms would create a separate and unequal college experience for women.

Chapter 4 explores how college hygiene departments gradually evolved from emphasizing physical education and sanitation into comprehensive health centers offering clinical care. Although preventive measures such as physical examinations and medical inspection of campus facilities became standard practice by the early 1900s, colleges and universities hesitated to establish clinics for students because they feared opposition from local physicians' groups, who were already disturbed by the spread of contract practice in factories, mining camps, and other industries. To address these concerns, college health professionals during the 1910s began a self-conscious effort to upgrade their field and establish special claims to knowledge that other physicians lacked. In 1920, physicians working in colleges and universities came together to form the American Student Health Association to share ideas and to establish networks for those engaged in college health work. At the same time, professionals in college health were influenced by the "new public health" of the early twentieth century, which focused on individual risk factors rather than broader environmental and social dangers. College health programs emphasized individual health care and hygiene education while downplaying the broader programs of sanitary reform that had characterized earlier public health efforts. This chapter argues that the professional legitimacy of college health as a field hinged partially on changing notions of about college students as a class of patients and the college environment as a locus for medical practice. During the early twentieth century, college health experts extended the adolescent status of semidependency into the young adult years, applying the concept to men as well as women. College physicians drew on the work of noted child psychologist G. Stanley Hall, who suggested that the college experience prolonged the adolescent stage of life. Emulating Hall, college physicians attempted to alleviate gender discrepancies in the regulation of campus life. Doctors argued that male students remained adolescents and therefore deserved the same protections in loco parentis as did their female counterparts.

Students played a central role in the growth of clinical services, as many found the free market of medical care in college communities beyond their means. Student demand for affordable medical care became especially strident at public universities. Those with limited resources found themselves forgoing medical care and/or dropping out of school entirely because of untreated health problems. In response, student organizations sought ways to finance health services for less fortunate students. Modeling themselves after insurance programs offered by fraternal organizations such as the Odd Fellows and Freemasons, some college organizations began in the early twentieth century to create health care funds for students who could not otherwise afford medical care. College physicians responded to these student-led initiatives by demonstrating the link between poor health and wastage of human potential. Drawing on examples from industrial medicine and the conservation movement, physicians argued that clinical services would help prepare student bodies to fit into the emerging industrial capitalist social order. They also claimed that college health services took the place of the family doctor and health supervision offered in students' own homes. This metaphor of the college infirmary as a surrogate home proved a successful strategy for parents. Students, however, did not usually share physicians' views about their ability to make mature health care decisions. Nevertheless, students compromised to obtain affordable and accessible health care.

The mainstream medical profession remained opposed to student health services as well as other forms of contract practice. Chapter 5 looks at how professionals in college health used links between student health and the health of the nation to further legitimize medical services for college students. This relationship between the fitness of the student body and the well-being of the body politic became especially prevalent in the 1930s and 1940s, as concerns about the strength of the United States as a world power intensified interest in preserving the health of the nation's student population. Although college students made up a small percentage of the young adult population throughout the twentieth century, college physicians argued that by virtue of their roles as future leaders and voters, protecting student bodies—in particular, male student bodies—was essential to the nation's viability. Disclosures about the poor health of college-aged military recruits during World Wars I and II as well as high rates of sexually transmitted diseases and tuberculosis among the college-aged population in 1920s and 1930s exacerbated existing fears about racial degeneration and provided yet another incentive for improving health services for college students. Physicians at both white institutions and historically black colleges and universities called for greater attention to black student health as part of a larger program of racial uplift. Physicians argued that college students, both black and white, could help sell hygiene to the American public, thereby elevating the status and cultural authority of the mainstream medical profession. These simultaneous efforts to "sell" college health programs by linking them to the nation's health culminated in the 1947 report of President Harry S. Truman's Commission on Higher Education, *Higher Education for American Democracy*, which stated that one of the major goals of higher education was to help improve the health of the individual student and thereby raise the standards of individual and community health throughout the nation. Although the mainstream medical profession remained opposed to Truman's attempts to establish national health insurance, the medical establishment became convinced that college health services, like other forms of prepaid group practice such as Kaiser Permanente, constituted a reasonable middle ground between traditional fee-for-service care and state-funded medical care.

Protection of the student body was not limited to physical health. Chapter 6 examines the emergence and development of mental hygiene programs for college and university students. Many professionals involved in student health services and student personnel work were inspired by the mental hygiene movement that began in the 1920s. Like their counterparts in elementary and secondary schools, college mental hygienists became interested in finding ways to prevent and treat mental disturbances in college students before they led to academic difficulties and failure. Student health services frequently worked in conjunction with departments of clinical psychology to study the incidence of emotional difficulty among the student body, as well as to design tests that would help predict which students would be most likely to experience maladjustments while in college. In the process, college health centers created psychological services that helped students manage the stresses of late adolescence and the academic and social pressures of college life. College mental hygiene experts also emphasized the importance of mental hygiene programs in fostering mature minds and healthy personalities among the nation's youth. Experts argued that giving students a greater role in college health programs formed a central part of promoting maturity and independence in college students.

This new commitment to a truly student-centered health service would have unintended consequences in the ensuing decade, as students rebelled against the paternalistic structure of American colleges and universities. Chapter 7 examines how student unrest in the 1960s and 1970s created new challenges for college health services. Throughout the 1960s, physicians and other health care professionals on college campuses became accustomed to treating students injured during protests as well as to fielding increasing requests for advice on birth control, sexuality, and the use of illegal drugs. Student leaders emulated the broader consumer rights movement by demanding a greater role in the services offered and in how their health fees were spent. Allied with other social movements of the 1960s and 1970s, such as the civil rights movement, women's liberation, gay rights, and disability rights, the student health activism during this period also led to more inclusive policies regarding race, physical appearance, and physical ability. During the 1970s, the American College Health Association recognized students' role in shaping health care by establishing the Student Advisory Committee to help shape the future of college health services. The student protests of the 1960s culminated in the abolition of parietal rules on most campuses. Unfortunately, student activism also prompted a backlash that reduced state allocations and institutional commitment to campus health programs that served "unruly" and "ungrateful" students. Faculty too criticized the medicalization of higher education by college health experts, especially those associated with psychiatry and student counseling.

The final chapter uses two recent health crises during the past two decades—the AIDS epidemic and the increase in mental health problems among students—to illustrate continuities and changes in college health over the past quarter century. The appearance of these and other dangers to student health has reopened discussions about the extent to which institutions of higher education are responsible for the health of their students. Members of the American College Health Association have used the new health risks faced by modern students to justify the ongoing need for college health programs emphasizing prevention and early intervention, especially given the escalating costs of medical care and the expanding ranks of uninsured and underinsured young adults. Notions about the relationship between the health of the student body and the health of the nation continue to play a major role in twenty-first-century health care debates. At the same time, the student movements of the 1960s and 1970s make a return to a paternalistic model of health promotion inappropriate, especially given that the fastest growing section of the student population falls beyond the traditional college age of eighteen to twenty-two and often has parental responsibilities of its own. Finding a balance between overly protective supervision and utter neglect continues to vex professionals concerned with the health of student bodies in the twenty-first century.

CHAPTER I

Educate a Woman and You Educate a Race

In January 2005, Harvard University president Lawrence H. Summers provoked a nationwide scandal when he suggested in a lecture at the National Bureau of Economic Research Conference that the dearth of women in science and engineering resulted from innate differences between the intellectual abilities of men and women. He also argued that women's traditional roles as wives and mothers conflicted with meeting the research expectations for faculty at Harvard and other elite universities. A protest letter from Harvard faculty charged that Summers's remarks sent "mixed signals" to the "high achieving women" at Harvard and other institutions of higher education.[1]

Since our nation's inception, ambivalence has existed about women's ability and need to pursue higher education. The political rhetoric of the Founding Fathers provided a major incentive for educating women. According to the ideology of republican motherhood, women played a critical role in ensuring that their children—particularly their sons—would acquire the civic virtue and intellectual skills vital to the health of the new nation.[2] Religious movements also provided a powerful justification for women's higher education. During the early nineteenth century, a nationwide religious revival known as the Second Great Awakening swept through the country and was especially popular among the nation's young people. Although few evangelical denominations granted women the full range of rights and responsibilities within the church, women's work was considered central to the larger cause of world salvation. Most denominations believed that Christian family values could not be taught to "heathens" unless male missionaries brought with them educated and pious wives. Women missionaries were also the only ones who could reach potential female converts in countries that observed strict sexual segregation. Women played a key role in religious work at home as well. By the mid–nineteenth century, women congregants far outnumbered men, and the missionary and outreach work of these organizations depended heavily on female voluntarism. The need to train women for missionary work both at home and abroad led to the creation of female seminaries such as Mount Holyoke in western Massachusetts and Troy Female Seminary in New York.[3]

As a result of these political and religious trends, educational institutions for girls and young women expanded greatly in the nineteenth century, thereby making U.S. women the most literate in the world. Although the curriculum at female institutions was quite rigorous for the time, they did not match the standards or the status of the elite men's colleges. Nevertheless, medical experts warned of the dangers that education posed to women's health. Numerous books and articles lamented the unhygienic conditions that prevailed at the majority of female institutions. For example, an article in the December 1837 *Boston Medical and Surgical Journal* exclaimed, "There is something radically wrong in the present system of education among young ladies. Their physical condition does not receive from parents or teachers that consideration which it deserves."[4] These concerns prompted female academies and seminaries to pay especially close attention to student health. At Mount Holyoke, for example, students were required to observe a strict schedule of prayer, study, meals, and exercise. The student handbook required all students to extinguish their lights at ten in the evening and leave their doors open so that the faculty could watch over them.[5]

In the 1870s, medical arguments against women's education were strengthened by the work of Harvard medical professor Dr. Edward Hammond Clarke, who warned of the dangers of higher education to the female brain and body in his best-selling book, *Sex in Education; or, A Fair Chance for the Girls* (1873). Drawing on the principle of the conservation of energy and notions of human evolution promoted by Charles Darwin and other naturalists, Clarke argued that the brain withdrew physical energy from the rest of the body during intellectual activities. Although Clarke acknowledged that such a mind-body linkage existed in both sexes, he contended that women's brains were less evolved than those of men. Furthermore, the unique characteristics of the female reproductive system made women more vulnerable to mental and physical breakdown. Energy depletion was especially treacherous during puberty, when the reproductive organs were still maturing. Even after puberty, Clarke claimed that women remained at risk for reproductive disorders and nervous ailments because of the disabilities caused by menstruation. Women who ignored these basic facts of nature by pursuing an education risked nervous collapse and sterility.[6]

These views did not go unchallenged. Prominent women reformers published scathing attacks on Clarke's work in the popular and medical press. The most widely read challenge to *Sex in Education* came from Dr. Mary Putnam Jacobi, a professor at the Women's Medical College of the New York Infirmary for Women and Children. In her landmark study, *The Question of Rest for Women during Menstruation* (1877), Jacobi published the results of a survey of the menstrual health of more than two hundred of her female patients. The responses she received led her to conclude, "There is nothing in the nature of menstruation to imply the necessity, or even the desirability, of rest, for women."[7] Even Clarke's colleagues recognized the importance of Jacobi's research, awarding her Harvard's prestigious Boylston Medical Prize in 1877.[8]

Jacobi was not alone in using science to undermine Clarke's claims, nor did this criticism come solely from female physicians and women's rights activists. Among the most noted male critics of Clarke's work was Nathan Allen, a widely respected member of the Massachusetts medical profession and a central figure in the commonwealth's nascent public health movement.[9] In his studies of population decline among prominent New England families, Allen observed "unmistakable signs of physical degeneracy" as well as other "startling facts" such as fewer marriages, lower birthrates, and growing numbers of divorces in this elite social group.[10] Unlike Clarke, however, Allen was part of a reform cohort who believed that all young people, not just women, were victims of an educational system that developed their minds at the expense of their bodies. In a lecture before the fiftieth annual meeting of the American Institute of Instruction in 1879, Allen argued that "if young men must depend for success in life upon the 'vigor of the body'" as well as the mind, then the same was true of women, who would go on to be "in the broadest and fullest sense the 'educators of the race.'"[11]

Despite these challenges, Clarke's ideas proved remarkably tenacious and seemed to be supported by the most advanced scientific evidence of the day. A large lay and scientific audience read Clarke's book, which sparked widespread discussion and criticism. The book proved so popular that it went through seventeen editions in thirteen years. Clarke's ideas captured the attention of Americans already anxious about conditions of modern life that they believed were undermining the health of the nation's young people. This feeling was particularly acute within the nation's growing cities, where crowded living conditions, sedentary work and school habits, and the hustle and bustle of daily urban life were thought to be creating a nation of flabby, nervous, mentally unstable, and physically diseased citizens. This growing sense of "dis-ease" in the body politic led to increased attention on the health of the physical body. Women were the primary target of nineteenth-century concerns about health and the future of the white race, as Clarke and other medical authorities alleged that female anatomy and physiology made women especially vulnerable to illness.[12]

Thus, despite the need to educate the race by educating mothers, the notion that women should receive a college education remained controversial. These anxieties about the fitness of the female body shaped the design of women's colleges and the female divisions of coeducational institutions. The earliest college health programs emerged to address concerns about the impact of higher education on the female body. These initiatives for women later served as models for further developments in college student health.

Better Than Gentleman's Schools of Kindred Grade

In 1865, wealthy industrialist Matthew Vassar announced his intention to endow "a College for young women which shall be to them, what Yale and Harvard are to young men."[13] Unlike most men of the day, Vassar and other founders of the college were progressive on the issue of women's intellectual abilities, believing that women's brains were no different from those of men. Thus, women deserved an equally demanding education. Clarke's jeremiad against women's higher education challenged this optimism because one of the six case studies mentioned in the book was allegedly a Vassar student. "Miss D" had entered the college in good health at the age of fourteen. As a result of a taxing academic schedule that matched that of a man, Miss D's health steadily declined during her junior and senior years at Vassar. She then graduated before nineteen "with fair honors and a poor physique." Clarke called this case yet "another text for the oft-repeated sermon on the delicacy of American girls." Rather than observing the laws of nature, the reproductive development is "shoved out of sight like a disgrace" in the ambition "to get what is popularly called an education."[14]

Vassar's resident physician, Alida C. Avery, quickly came to the college's defense. In an impassioned letter to Clarke, Avery argued for the unfairness of assuming from one case that ill health in women college students resulted from advanced study. Yet Avery also underscored the zealous precautions she and her colleagues at Vassar took to prevent tragedies like that of Miss D. The college's rural setting and campus buildings were designed to ensure complete control over students' minds and bodies. The college employed a "lady principal" who closely supervised the personal habits of the students. Because there were few effective medical therapies at this time, medical experts and laypersons alike believed that the best way to preserve health was to prevent diseases before they started. Popular health manuals at this time espoused theories that suggested that disease resulted from a combination of constitutional irregularities inherited from one's ancestors, poor living habits, and an unsanitary environment. Of these three factors, health advice writers considered individual behavior to be the most malleable. They therefore encouraged their readers to engage in regular exercise, get adequate rest, eat sensible diets, and abstain from alcohol, tobacco, and other stimulating substances.[15]

Physical education was central to protecting student health at Vassar, since medical opinion at this time stated that physical fitness was the best way to prevent disease and debility. The first student handbook for the college noted that physical education is "*fundamental* to all the rest."[16] Vassar employed the exercise system promoted by Boston health reformer and physical education instructor Dio Lewis. Lewis's system of "light gymnastics," based on similar programs in Sweden and Germany, involved calisthenics with light dumbbells and other apparatus. Lewis's textbook, *New Gymnastics for Men, Women, and Children* (1862) went through ten editions and became a standard text for many schools, colleges, and homes. According to Lewis, moderate physical exercise as well as other personal habits such as avoidance of alcohol, regular bathing, good diet, and adequate rest and relaxation were remedies for the neurasthenia, or nervous exhaustion, that plagued students and other sedentary "brain workers" of the mid–nineteenth century. Lewis was also an ardent supporter of women's rights, claiming that regular exercise and dress reform were vital to improving the physical and social status of American women.[17]

Likewise, Avery claimed that her primary aim was "to combine opportunity for serious mental activity with physical training and individual freedom from tiresome restraint" imposed by corsets and other restrictive clothing. Avery hoped "vigor of head and heart and body will be the happy result."[18] Indeed, she asserted that the regimen at Vassar not only preserved but actually improved the students' health. In her practice at the college, Avery observed numerous students "who came to us weak, indifferent, listless, full of morbid whims and uncontrolled caprices of mind and body." After spending four years in Vassar's "bracing atmosphere of happy, sustained industry," these sickly girls gained "such an impetus toward real health that they forgot aches and discontents, and went home ready and eager to do their share in the world's work."[19]

Of course, some students often found these restrictions and requirements excessive. One student complained in 1868 that the "only trouble here is they won't let us study enough. . . . They are afraid we shall break down." Nevertheless, this student realized that the "reputation of the college is at stake, for the question is can girls get a college degree without injuring their health?"[20]

Such concerns were not limited to Vassar College. Because the other Seven Sisters were founded in the midst of the controversy surrounding Clarke's book, administrators at these newer women's colleges had little choice but to pay close attention to student bodies. Like the officials at Vassar, other schools' founders and administrators believed that a woman's education should be as thorough and demanding as a man's but also realized that extra provisions should be made for women students because of their fragile health. Martha Carey Thomas, president of Bryn Mawr, acknowledged that when the college first opened in the 1880s, she was uncertain "whether women's health could stand the strain of education. We were haunted in those days by the clanging chains of that gloomy little specter, Dr. Edward Clarke's *Sex in Education*."[21] President Alice Freeman Palmer of Wellesley College (founded in 1875) claimed that while "the chief business of a man's college . . . is to give instruction of the best available quality in as many subjects as possible," the aim of the woman's college was "to do all this but . . . also provide for its students a home within its own walls" and accept the "responsibility not only of the present health of its students, but also in large degree of their physical power in the future."[22]

Administrators, physicians, and physical educators at the women's colleges founded after 1875 looked for new ways to assure that their women students were both well educated and able-bodied. In 1875, Smith College introduced a new system of student housing designed to emulate the late-Victorian home. Smith's founders also believed that a cottage system would control the spread of epidemic diseases that swept through larger dormitories at this time. Noting the improved healthfulness of this new housing system, a writer for the *Ladies' Home Journal* observed, "Nowhere did I find girls more bright, healthful, and comfortable than at Smith College."[23] Eager to compete for students, officials at the older residential women's colleges imitated the housing innovations made in Northampton.[24]

One sees this concern about protecting female bodies even at Radcliffe, where the founders originally opposed any buildings or regulations that would replicate what trustees believed to be the "unnatural" and "convent-like" conditions of the residential women's colleges. Nevertheless, early annual reports made certain to mention that the health of the young ladies was excellent and in some cases had actually improved. Although there were no dormitories, the college required students to live in houses approved by a committee of women appointed by the Radcliffe Corporation. Students could not board with families where Harvard students lived, although the college allowed Radcliffe students to reside in the same boardinghouses as Harvard faculty. The trustees argued that placing students in families was particularly important for younger and less mature students, for it provided them the "protections of home" and ensured "regularity of life and propriety of behavior."[25]

Radcliffe officials closely adhered to the advice of renowned Philadelphia neurologist S. Weir Mitchell, who claimed that many of the female health problems he observed in his practice resulted from the mental and physical strain of higher education. In an address to the graduating class of Radcliffe College, Mitchell stated that while he did not entirely oppose collegiate education for women, he also believed that "if the higher education or the college life in any way, body or mind, unfits women to be good wives and mothers there had better be none of it." Mitchell praised women's colleges that employed physicians to "prevent disaster by due regulation of work, play, diet, exercise, and the inhibition of mind-labor when physiology and reason forbid it."[26] Following this example, Radcliffe College constructed a lunchroom and a gymnasium for students in the 1890s and hired Dr. Henry P. Walcott as medical adviser in 1893.[27] By 1898, Radcliffe graduates realized that the lack of campus housing was working against the college. That year, the alumnae and the Annex '95 club began to raise money for a residence hall system "carefully limited in size, healthful, tasteful, economical and bearing the prestige of college ownership," which would offer all Radcliffe students, regardless of income, the "essentials, physical, aesthetic and social as well as intellectual, of a true College education." The desire to reassure parents from outside the Boston area that their daughters would be adequately protected while in

Cambridge eventually led to the construction of Bertram Hall, Radcliffe's first dormitory, in 1905.[28]

To demonstrate the effectiveness of their programs on the female body, physicians and physical educators at the women's colleges drew on the new science of anthropometry, or the measurement of human growth. The systematic study of human characteristics grew partly out of the work of the eighteenth-century French encyclopedists, who incorporated the study of human morphology and racial variation into their studies of the natural world. French scientists alleged that the American environment stunted the growth of its inhabitants. As evidence, the French gave reports of the supposed inferior stature and morphology of Native Americans as well as African slaves and white settlers. Eager to disprove these erroneous claims, early American naturalists, including Thomas Jefferson and Benjamin Franklin, collected data that showed that American plants, animals, and humans were equal or even superior to their European counterparts. The work of Belgian mathematician Lambert A. J. Quetelet also had a central role in developing the science of anthropometry. Originally trained as an astronomer, Quetelet extended the principles of mathematics to the study of human beings and social institutions. He hoped that by discerning the laws of human behavior he could help solve such intractable social problems as crime, suicide, and poverty. Quetelet's notion of the "average man" gained great currency both in Europe and the United States, and his book, *A Treatise on Man and the Development of His Faculties* (1835), became the standard work for other researchers in the field.[29]

Physicians and physical educators at the women's colleges extended these observations, finding that American college women were healthier, taller, and stronger than women from the same ethnic and economic background who did not attend college. Supporters claimed that by producing healthier, more physically fit, and better-educated mothers, women's colleges would make the white race that much stronger and wiser.[30] The most prominent proponent of this idea that physical education for women contributed to race betterment was Dudley Allen Sargent, who directed the Hemenway Gymnasium at Radcliffe. Sargent observed that the intellectual advancement of the white upper classes had led to larger head size and argued that "unless the woman's body is perfectly developed to meet this condition, it means her immolation and the deterioration of the race." Sargent further claimed that physical education could remedy this problem by enlarging women's pelvises and ensuring that their bodies were fit for reproduction.[31] He also drew on the work of noted neurologist Edward Seguin, who believed that "feeblemindedness" in children and nervous ailments in adults were caused by a degeneration of the nervous system that could be alleviated by training the body's muscles and nerves. Seguin's work convinced Sargent of the importance of physical activity in education. To prove his theories, Sargent set up a hygienic institute in New York City, designed to build the bodies of men, women, and children "who were naturally weak, or who had run down in the race of human endeavor."[32]

Sargent believed that foreign systems of gymnastics, such as those espoused by Lewis, were insufficient for combating the stress and strain of modern life. Instead, he used data compiled from his own anthropometric studies to devise appliances and exercise systems that ensured symmetrical development of the body. The Sargent system consisted of more than fifty tests of size and strength of different parts of the body, conducted with tape measures, spring dynameters, and other devices designed and built by Sargent and his staff. After gathering data on more than ten thousand women, Sargent prepared standardized charts against which he measured individual students. For those who did not meet these standards, Sargent designed a personalized exercise program aimed at correcting specific physical defects and improving overall physical fitness.[33]

Sargent promoted his system in numerous scientific and popular articles and set up a normal school to train male and female teachers in his methods. The other women's colleges were so impressed with Sargent's work at Radcliffe that they soon hired his female normal school graduates to implement similar programs on their campuses. These women physical educators duplicated Sargent's findings. At Wellesley, Lucille Eaton Hill and her assistant, M. Anna Wood, collected statistics on nearly two thousand students that demonstrated the positive impact of exercise on the female physique. This data became a central piece of Wellesley's promotional literature. An article in the *American Review of Reviews* claimed that Wellesley led the way in making college a "place where the health of young women is sedulously and scientifically guarded, and where her physical strength and well-being are systematically developed."[34] President Anna J. MacKeag of Wilson College for Women in Chambersburg, Pennsylvania, observed that a "more vigorous and active body of women than those of our colleges it would be hard to find anywhere," given the favorable conditions present at the women's colleges.[35] Students also testified to the benefits of the carefully supervised physical exercise they received in college. For example, Sophia Foster Richardson, a Vassar alumna, said she owed her good health since graduation to the "regularity of college life and to vigorous play" and could therefore could not understand the perspective of those who opposed women's higher education.[36]

In 1885, the Association of College Alumnae, forerunner of the American Association of University Women, published a survey claiming that the college environment was more conducive to female health than other occupations. Although 19.58 percent of the alumnae respondents complained of a deterioration of health while in college, 21.13 reported improvement. Annie G. Howes, chair of the committee in charge of compiling the statistics, exclaimed that she was "confident that a higher education for women is in harmony with that vast law of the survival of the fittest which guides the activities of the dim future."[37]

Amherst College physician and hygiene professor Dr. Edward Hitchcock Jr. echoed these opinions. After examining a comparison of mortality statistics of Mount Holyoke graduates with those of male colleges made in the late 1860s, Hitchcock found that the mortality rate among male college students, excluding Civil War casualties, was higher than that of female students. Hitchcock concluded that women's colleges not only instilled high levels of scholarship and religious culture but also produced a "health-influence [that] holds out better than in gentlemen's schools of kindred grade."[38]

Yet the controversy over female higher education precipitated by Clarke's book was far from over. Indeed, Clarke's supporters received additional ammunition with the publication of G. Stanley Hall's epic 1904 study on adolescence. "That woman can do many things as well as man does not prove that she ought to do the same things, or that man-made ways are the best for her," Hall argued. Although he did not completely oppose female higher education, he was alarmed by data indicating that graduates of women's colleges were less likely to marry and have children than those who had not attended college. Hall concluded that the health of the woman was "even more important for the welfare of the race than that of man." Institutions charged with educating girls in their teens and twenties, "when the period most favorable to motherhood begins," should emulate the "cult of the goddess Hygeia" by requiring students to follow the latest recommendations in nutrition, sleep, exercise, and other advances in "health culture."[39] These warnings about the dangers of higher education on the female body would shape coeducational institutions just as they had the women's colleges before them.

Women's Health and the Limits of Coeducation

Between 1860 and 1900, higher education opportunities for women gained ground with the tremendous growth of public schools. The need to educate children in western settlements, those of recent immigrants, and freed slaves created a desperate need for a cheap and plentiful teaching force. Educational reformers such as Catharine Beecher reiterated the doctrine of republican motherhood, proclaiming that educating children was the "true and noble profession of a woman." Moreover, school districts favored female teachers because women would accept lower salaries than would men. As new occupational opportunities opened for men in business, industry, and other professions, public school teaching evolved from a job of last resort for men to a profession for which women were considered eminently suited. To meet the need for trained teachers, states created normal schools that provided a shorter period of training at a lower cost than did private colleges.[40]

Other higher education options for women expanded as well. Elite private colleges and universities such as Cornell and the University of Chicago also opened to women, although reluctantly in many cases. State-funded education grew tremendously following the Morrill Land Grant Act (1862), which made public lands available to endow colleges for training in agriculture and the mechanical arts. Although the act did not require that women be admitted to the new state institutions, it also did not forbid their entrance. Some state universities resisted coeducation, while others admitted women rather than using additional funds to create separate female institutions. Elite male colleges remained closed to women, but some created coordinate female colleges such as Barnard (Columbia), Douglas (Rutgers), and Pembroke (Brown). By 1900, the United States had fifty-six thousand female college students, a fivefold increase since the end of the Civil War.[41]

Like the older women's colleges, these newer institutions were forced to address concerns about the impact of higher education on the female body. Amenities for women students frequently were prompted by economic concerns. For example, when Cornell first opened, the women's dormitory, Sage College, did not have a chaperone or matron during its first years of operation. By 1879, the university was in desperate economic circumstances as male enrollment declined and female enrollment failed to close the gap. Because of its nondenominational status, Cornell constantly faced accusations of being a "godless institution," and parents preferred sending their children to institutions that would instill proper Christian (usually Protestant) values. Administrators speculated that parents were especially reluctant to send their daughters to Cornell because of the "freedom and potential of moral dangers" at Sage College. Therefore, during the late nineteenth century, the university continually looked for ways to improve its popular image. Despite protests from women students about the "iron boarding house rules" that would accompany supervision, the board of trustees hired a matron to oversee the students in Sage. The board also made "every possible provision to ensure the health of [Sage's] inhabitants" by providing them with comfortable beds, nourishing food, well-ventilated rooms, modern bathroom facilities with indoor plumbing, and mandatory lectures on physiology and hygiene. In 1884, the university declared that all women students must reside in the dormitory. Women who did not wish to comply with this requirement were dismissed from the university, since the trustees believed it would be better for women to be forgo a college education than to "undermine their constitutions" through advanced study.[42]

This transition was not unique to Cornell: by the early twentieth century, many other private coeducational institutions had begun regulating female students' living arrangements as a way of reassuring parents that their daughters' physical and moral welfare would be safeguarded. Small coeducational institutions such as Grinnell and Carleton built residence halls where women could be segregated from male students.[43] The University of Chicago provided dormitories for women when it first opened in 1892. When dean of women Marion Talbot discovered that most students could not afford to reside on campus, she urged the university to protect women from the city's physical and social ills by creating a housing department to inspect the physical condition of boardinghouses and, more importantly, make sure that male and female students did not share the same residences. Talbot also strictly policed student behavior, insisting that women uphold respectable standards of dress, conduct, and manners. She also forbade smoking, drinking, and other "dangerous habits" in the women's dormitories. In 1915, a generous gift from Laverne Noyes enabled the university to construct Ida Noyes Hall, which contained clubrooms, a gymnasium, a swimming pool, and lunchrooms, all of which helped the university more closely supervise the health habits of female students.[44]

Other elite colleges were unwilling to provide services for girls and young women in loco parentis, instead using concerns about the effects of higher education on female health to limit or deny women's admission. For example, at the University of Pennsylvania, women students were permitted to be "special students" in the Towne Scientific School beginning in the 1870s, but few were allowed to study in the other graduate and professional schools. After the opening of the School of Education in 1914, women were allowed to receive bachelor's degrees in the normal program in education. Women were excluded from the undergraduate college until 1933, partly because of fears about how education would affect their health but also because administrators wanted to preserve the university's prestige relative to other all-male colleges.[45]

State institutions did not have the same leeway. As "people's colleges" funded by state tax dollars, the public normal schools and land-grant colleges founded in the mid- to late nineteenth century had to take all qualified applicants. Most states found it too costly to build separate colleges for women. In addition, the desperate need for public school teachers in the years following the Civil War made rejection of female applicants impractical.[46]

Single-sex public institutions were more common in the southeastern states, as were separate institutions for African Americans. Indeed, women's educational opportunities in the South actually declined after the Civil War, as state governments in the former Confederacy lacked sufficient funds to rebuild public colleges damaged or destroyed by warfare. Even before the war, advanced study was limited to daughters of the wealthy, planter elite, and higher education for southern women was intended to prepare them for their roles as decorative plantation wives and mothers. The expansion of public schooling during Reconstruction as well as a need to provide "respectable" employment for widows and daughters of Confederate soldiers led to the creation of public normal schools in many southeastern states. Yet these institutions were poorly funded and offered a shorter course of study than the four-year state research and technical universities, which remained closed to women.[47]

Like private universities, these public institutions had to contend with the warnings about the negative impact of higher education on female health. This was especially true at state normal schools, which realized that the health of future teachers was essential for their larger mission of improving school hygiene.[48] This concern with the health of female normal school students is illustrated by the history of Framingham State Normal School. Established in Lexington in 1839 and moved to Framingham in 1853, the normal school was the first publicly funded teacher training institution in the Commonwealth of Massachusetts. Since the female students came from the surrounding area, school officials did not believe it necessary to provide housing for them. Yet Framingham employed a female physician, Mary J. Studley, to oversee student health. Following her graduation from Framingham State in 1852, Studley worked as a public school teacher in Massachusetts. She obtained a medical degree from the New York Infirmary for Women and Children in 1872 and was appointed resident physician and teacher of natural sciences at Framingham in 1877. Like her counterparts at the women's colleges, Studley believed that the best way to alleviate the nervous strain caused by advanced study was a "well-developed muscular system." Studley found that the majority of young women schoolteachers she observed were "notably deficient" in this area. She therefore believed that only women who developed sufficient strength and physical stamina for enduring the rigors of the classroom should be allowed to become teachers.[49]

Studley's reputation at Framingham State soon led to requests from both students and their mothers for written copies of the lectures she gave at the normal school. The resulting volume, *What Our Girls Ought to Know* (1878), was extremely popular and went through several editions. In her introduction, Studley observed that her experience with Framingham students "convinces me that they do not willfully sin against their bodies, but are sadly ignorant of the laws which govern them." While instruction in hygiene traditionally had been a mother's duty, "it is a lamentable fact that the present generation of mothers is woefully deficient in the ability to do so." Indeed, she claimed that mothers were "glad to secure the aid of an educated lady physician in supplementing their home work."[50]

Other institutions of higher education were also eager to employ "lady physicians" to protect the female student body. The position of college physician and/or professor of hygiene and physiology soon became one of the few professional opportunities for female physicians in the late nineteenth and early twentieth centuries.[51] The earliest faculty positions for women at coeducational institutions typically involved supervising physical training and/or teaching courses in hygiene.[52] Administrative opportunities for professional women also evolved out of the duties of women physicians appointed to oversee the health of and morality of female students at coeducational institutions. At the University of California at Berkeley, the first female administrator was Dr. Mary Ritter, who served as both physician and unofficial overseer of campus life for women undergraduates.[53]

Like their predecessors at the women's colleges, physicians at coeducational institutions conducted anthropometric studies of their students to confirm that college life, and physical education in particular, improved rather than damaged women's bodies. Among the most notable studies were those conducted by Dr. Clelia Duel Mosher, physician and professor in the department of hygiene at Stanford University. Mosher used her experiences as a child and young woman to illustrate the importance of exercise and physiological knowledge for women students. Mosher had been so sickly as a child that her father attempted to keep her out of college. Nevertheless, she found the financial resources and physical strength to attend Wellesley College. Although ill health and the death of her father forced her to drop out after two years, she went on to obtain degrees in zoology and physiology from the University of Wisconsin and was among the first women graduates of the Johns Hopkins University Medical School. After receiving her M.D. in 1900, Mosher worked as an intern in gynecology. In 1910, finding most other employment options closed to her, Mosher accepted an appointment as assistant professor of personal hygiene, medical adviser for women, and director of the Roble Gymnasium at Stanford.[54]

In addition to her official duties, Mosher continued her interest in anatomy and physiology and invented a device called a schematograph to study posture and changes in bodily proportions.[55] She observed from results gathered over a period of thirty years that the heights, weights, and overall physical health of female students had improved over the course of her career at Stanford. "The racial as well as economic importance of these changes, which point to a more fully developed and more perfectly functioning type of woman, can hardly be overestimated," wrote Mosher in a 1921 article.[56] Mosher also gathered data on her students' menstrual periods, noting that while some women had severe menstrual cramps, for most women menstruation was in no way a disabling condition. She also believed that exercise could greatly alleviate menstrual pain and developed a system of exercises aimed at reducing the duration of and discomfort associated with periods.[57] Some students complained about doing their daily "moshers" and were dismayed that they could no longer use their menstrual periods to get out of gymnasium exercises or other classes. Others considered Mosher's system a godsend. One student told her, "You should be canonized for inventing these menstrual exercises."[58] Another student wrote to Mosher that her freshman hygiene class was "invaluable" as "my whole life has been enriched by it."[59]

Mosher popularized her results and their implications in her books, *Health and the Woman Movement* (1916) and *Woman's Physical Freedom* (1923). Both books undercut the physiological arguments that had been used to deny women access to higher education. Mosher declared that the college woman approached the "old Greek ideal of physical perfection" and was the "mother of finer sons and daughters, the promise of a stronger race. This same achievement is now possible for all women," Mosher promised, as long as they followed the same laws of hygiene imposed on women in college.[60]

Prominent female academics hailed Mosher's work as being as significant as that of Mary Putnam Jacobi a generation earlier.[61] Mosher's studies also deeply impressed some male scientists. Havelock Ellis, for example, wrote to her that he was "greatly interested in your preliminary note of investigations on normal menstruation as your observations belong to a class of evidence which I am very anxious to obtain."[62] Even Hall grudgingly admitted, "I wish very much that your work had come to my notice in season to be noted in the *Adolescence.* It seems to me very highly desirable that you should continue and complete these studies, for this seems to me one of the most important of all topics for hygiene, education and for the future of the race."[63]

Yet heightened attention to women's bodies caused significant disparities between male and female campus life. The history of women's experiences at the University of Michigan shows how campus policies created a segregated college experience for women. When women students first were admitted to Michigan in 1870, they, like male students, were allowed to live off campus in boardinghouses without any sort of supervision or provision for health. As Cornell and other coeducational institutions began to provide health supervision and regulations to women students in loco parentis, however, Michigan found that it had to do likewise to compete for the best students. In 1895, University of Michigan president James Burrill Angell appointed Michigan graduate Eliza Mosher (M.D. 1875) to the position of dean of women, which included oversight of the gymnasium, physical education, and courses in hygiene and sanitary science. Although women and men continued to share boardinghouses off campus, only women were subject to parietals, and women faced discipline for entertaining men in their rooms. In the late 1890s, a group of faculty wives formed the Michigan League to ensure that certain approved boardinghouses rented only to women and set aside public parlors for male visitors. By 1900, the league began a campaign to build women's dormitories that would ensure even more administrative oversight over female students' well-being.[64]

The University of California was slower to institute similar protections for women students, largely because the institution was not fully committed to coeducation. The university did not build dormitories for either women or men until the 1920s. Because boardinghouse keepers frequently doubted the respectability of single females seeking housing on their own, many preferred to rent their rooms exclusively to men. Consequently, men found it easier to locate lodging close to campus, and women had no choice but to endure long commutes. This situation compelled some families to move to Berkeley rather than allow their daughters to make the daily trek across the bay. Not until the appointment of Phoebe Apperson Hearst as the first woman regent of the University of California in 1891 did the campus lives of Berkeley women receive more serious attention, although it frequently resulted from the students' activism. In 1898, the regents permitted Hearst to fund the part-time appointment of Dr. Mary Bennett Ritter as physician to women students and lecturer in hygiene.[65] Ritter had previously been serving as an informal health adviser to female students. Her husband, William, was head of Berkeley's zoology department, and as a prominent faculty wife and one of the few female physicians in the area, Ritter became a trusted adviser for many female students. When the director of Harmon Gymnasium refused to allow women students to use the facility without first obtaining medical examinations, Ritter offered to do so free of charge on top of her thriving private practice. Ritter's appointment as a part-time faculty member allowed her to keep regular office hours for students every morning, "where girls could consult me about their ills of body, mind or 'hearts.'" Ritter also found that "many of the young women were seriously interested in their physical well-being and wished to know more about themselves and about home-making." These requests led Ritter to offer lectures in home sanitation and personal hygiene, which eventually became part of a mandatory hygiene course for first-year women. Since Ritter was often the only woman on the campus to whom the girls could turn for any personal advice, demand for both medical services and individual help grew tremendously. Students frequently asked Ritter for assistance in locating affordable room and board. Ritter found "malnutrition common among them and knew that many were skimping too severely." Ritter also persuaded Berkeley president Benjamin Ide Wheeler to allow her to inspect local boardinghouses and prevent students from living in residences that did not comply with the city's sanitary regulations by connecting to public water and sewage systems. Ritter added that regular inspection would also ensure that men and women did not reside in the same houses. Ritter recalled that during her years at Berkeley, "on a few occasions hasty marriages were arranged after too ardent love-making, but the standard of morality was very high." When Ritter reported to Hearst that many female students still lived in rather dismal circumstances, Hearst agreed to pay for Ritter to visit eastern women's colleges and coeducational institutions such as Cornell, Chicago, and Wisconsin to see how these institutions oversaw student life on and off campus. Upon her return to Berkeley in the summer of 1900, Ritter persuaded Hearst to furnish women's clubhouses to be run like the Smith cottage system, providing "respectable, attractive housing for women, without the social elitism of sororities." When Hearst left Berkeley in 1900, she donated her home to the university to be used as a women's gymnasium, thereby enabling the university to make physical education mandatory for all female students.[66]

Colleges and universities for African American women also designed their campuses to protect female student health. Prior to the Civil War, few higher education options existed for African Americans, male or female. Oberlin College took a huge financial risk when it decided to include African American students among its first entering class in 1833. This commitment to racial equality alienated all but the staunchest abolitionists, as most parents and students preferred institutions that did not permit mixing of the races.[67] Only two historically black colleges—Lincoln University in Pennsylvania and Wilberforce University in Ohio—were founded prior to the Civil War. Discrimination continued after the war, as northern colleges admitted only a handful of African Americans and southern institutions remained closed to blacks altogether. During Reconstruction, various denominational groups and freedman's aid societies established secondary schools, normal schools, and colleges for blacks in the former Confederacy. Funding from the federal government and northern philanthropists such as Julius Rosenwald and John D. Rockefeller also helped fuel the growth of black educational institutions in the United States. Although most of these institutions focused on the model of industrial education advocated by Booker T. Washington, a few had higher aspirations to educate an elite who would help uplift the standing of the black race as a whole. Although the cost of college remained beyond the means of most black families, the number of African Americans attending high school and college increased significantly between 1870 and 1915.[68]

Some African Americans, like whites, nonetheless remained ambivalent about whether black women should receive the same education as men. When Livingstone College opened in Salisbury, North Carolina, in 1880, some African American parents felt the institution went too far in its attempts to provide equal educational opportunities for men and women. These parents were also concerned about the propriety of coeducation. Instead, they adopted white gender norms of this period, preferring to send their daughters to single-sex religious institutions. Livingstone officials responded to these concerns by severely curtailing socialization between male and female students.[69]

Segregation in housing and medical care prompted black women's colleges to build dormitories and infirmaries for their students. Administrators were especially concerned with protecting female students, given the long history of black women's sexual victimization by white men. Officials at Spelman College not only provided a healthful environment but also ensured that students adopted respectable middle-class health habits. By following advice on hygiene and deportment, Spelman students "thus displayed not only better health but also a more refined, orderly, Christian way of life."[70]

Thus, to paraphrase Hitchcock's remarks about the women's colleges, when it came to matters of health, the female divisions of coeducational institutions as well as institutions for female African American students were better than white men's institutions of similar quality. This did not mean that white men's institutions were unenlightened; rather, the focus on protecting women's bodies and minds reflected widely held beliefs about the physical and mental characteristics of the "weaker sex." Even the most progressive educators of the day tended to reinforce this model of female anatomy and physiology, which tied the fitness of women's bodies and minds to the future of the race. Concerns about race suicide and racial degeneration would surface in discussions about the health of college men, serving to justify the development of hygiene programs aimed at building their bodies along with their brains.

CHAPTER 2

Building Manly Bodies and Moral Minds

In a report to the Amherst College board of trustees in 1855, newly appointed president William Augustus Stearns declared, "No one thing has demanded more of my anxious attention than the health of the students." Stearns observed numerous cases of students who had broken down, left school, or met untimely deaths while at college. He blamed the students' failing health on the sedentary life of the scholar, during which "physical exercise is neglected, the laws of health are violated, the protests and exhortations of instructors and other friends are unheeded." Stearns told the trustees that the circumstances of campus life at Amherst called for "immediate and efficient action."[1]

Stearns was not the first to suggest that regular exercise could protect the male body from physical and moral ills. In his proposal to create the institution that would eventually become the University of Pennsylvania, Benjamin Franklin wrote in 1749 that the masters should "look on the students as in some sort their children." Franklin argued that to keep students healthy, their bodies should be "frequently exercised in running, leaping, wrestling, and swimming."[2] However, these recommendations less reflected contemporary medical theory than embodied the paternalism of early American colleges. Both the curriculum and the daily life of colonial colleges were modeled after European universities that were born in the Middle Ages and therefore imposed on their students a medieval model of monastic discipline and piety.[3] Moreover, exercise programs for students were desultory at best and were based on the recommendations of colonial physician Benjamin Rush that the "amusements of our youth shall consist of such exercises as will be most subservient to their future employments in life." Colleges found that they could provide opportunities for physical activity and save money at the same time by requiring their students to perform various chores around the campus. Some even had working farms that generated additional income for the institution, as was the case with Oberlin College. Others provided charity students with land to cultivate to raise funds to pay for tuition, room, and board. During the 1820s, some colleges began to construct gymnasia, usually at the request of students and alumni, who raised funds for such structures. Students were free to use the facilities whenever they wanted without formal instruction or oversight but were seldom required to exercise.[4]

What set Amherst apart was the level of commitment the college showed to establishing physical education and hygiene as a legitimate academic discipline. In 1859, Stearns, along with trustees Henry Ward Beecher, Dr. Nathan Allen, and Dr. Ebenezer Alden, began a campaign to raise funds for Barrett Gymnasium, completed in 1860 and named in honor of chief benefactor Dr. Benjamin Barrett. In addition to creating a gymnasium, as had other colleges at the time, Stearns asked the trustees to raise an endowment for a professorship of hygiene and physical education. He also suggested that physical training and hygiene instruction be made a regular, required part of the curriculum. In 1860, the trustees appointed Dr. J. W. Hooker, a graduate of Yale Medical School, to direct the physical education program. Hooker resigned a few months later because of ill health and was replaced by Dr. Edward Hitchcock Jr., an Amherst alumnus and graduate of Harvard Medical School.[5]

According to Allen's recollections, these events constituted a landmark in the history of physical education, as it was the first time in the history of men's modern higher education "where the claims of the body, its proper development and healthy training, have been placed upon the same platform, and the same importance attached to them as to any other branch of study or mental acquirement."[6] Given Allen's position as trustee for Amherst College, a bit of skepticism about these grandiose claims is warranted. However, even Amherst's competitors admitted that the college led the way in its dedication to physical education as an academic discipline. As President Charles W. Eliot of Harvard remarked in 1880, "It is to Amherst College that the colleges of the country are indebted for a demonstration of the proper mode of organizing the department of physical training." Eliot declared that only Amherst had "established this department on the right basis, by putting it into the hands of an educated physician." Nearly two decades would pass before the other men's colleges emulated Amherst's example.[7]

Since the late nineteenth century, the notion that Amherst College provided the model for other college health programs has become accepted wisdom, particularly among professionals involved in college health. As the previous chapter showed, however, the women's colleges led the way in protecting student health, a fact that Hitchcock himself acknowledged. This situation would soon change, as new standards of public health and social attitudes focused increased attention on building male student bodies.

The Amherst Way; or, A Fair Chance for the Boys

Like many other men's colleges established in the early years of the new nation, Amherst proved fertile ground for the religious enthusiasm and reform sentiments of antebellum America. From its inception, Amherst was dedicated primarily to preparing young men for the ministry, thereby attracting young men who were driven by a "passionate desire to become clergymen." Foremost among Amherst's illustrious early graduates was Henry Ward Beecher (1834), brother of Harriet Beecher Stowe and the most renowned minister of his time. Accounts of college life during this period describe "zealous students" who spent "whole days together in fasting and prayer." To be sure, Amherst experienced its share of youthful indiscretions, as not all students arrived at the college with such a strong sense of religious conviction. Nevertheless, revivalism "spread quickly, and conversions were reported daily."[8]

This religious ethic affected the faculty as well. Most notable was Professor Edward Hitchcock Sr., father of the future hygiene director, who exemplified the connection between evangelical Christianity and public health reform. Originally trained as a Congregational minister, the elder Hitchcock became enamored with natural history. Despite his lack of a college degree, he was appointed professor of chemistry and natural history in 1825, later serving as the college's president from 1845 to 1854. Hitchcock was also an ardent temperance advocate, an interest driven in part by his own recurrent health problems. The senior Hitchcock was instrumental in establishing an Antivenean Society dedicated to stamping out the consumption of alcohol, tobacco, narcotics, and other "poisons."[9] A chronic sufferer of dyspepsia, Hitchcock also lectured extensively to students on the evils of gluttony, which he believed contributed to the "premature prostration and early decay of students and professional men in our country." Hitchcock regarded Americans' excessive consumption of meat as especially dangerous. Most at risk were students, professional men, and other sedentary persons for whom "the effect of such animal food is to produce too much excitement in the system, and to urge on the powers of life too fast."[10] This euphemistic language alluded to the sexual activities of the young men who were moving to the nation's cities and larger towns for employment. A flourishing and highly visible sex trade grew to serve the sexual appetites of these young men living independently of parental or adult supervision. Drawing on ancient humoral theory, medical experts at this time claimed that semen was a bodily fluid essential to the maintenance of both physical and mental health. Depletion of this fluid through the "solitary vice" as well as nocturnal emissions, fornication, adultery, and even excessive sexual intercourse within marriage could lead to a host of physical and mental ills, including tuberculosis, myopia, and insanity. Medical authorities in the nineteenth century used metaphors of the growing American capitalist system, describing a "spermatic economy" in which semen was likened to a bank account that could be depleted through excessive, frequent withdrawals. Physicians and parents alike were especially alarmed about masturbation in children and adolescents, since the age between onset of puberty and age of marriage widened markedly in the nineteenth century, especially for offspring of the middle class. Popular health advice literature advocated mental discipline and regular physical activity as a way to divert boys and young men from this noxious habit. In addition, the practice of circumcising non-Jewish males was first introduced as a method of dealing with the most intractable cases.[11]

Although the senior Hitchcock stopped short of advocating strict vegetarianism, he did suggest that sedentary brain workers "should not use animal food more than once a day." He was also an avid proponent of regular physical exercise, remarking that the exhilaration produced during his geological expeditions "has made me forgetful of my real or fancied ailments, and even expelled the nervousness and gloom of dyspeptic, bronchial, and neuralgic attacks."[12]

The elder Hitchcock's piety and commitment to health reform profoundly affected his son, who graduated from Amherst and chose to pursue a career in medicine. After receiving his medical degree from Harvard in 1853, the younger Hitchcock traveled with his brother-in-law, Pixlee Judson, to study at clinics and hospitals in Paris and London, considered the forefront of research and anatomy and physiology at this time. Hitchcock's scientific studies culminated at the British Museum in the laboratory of Sir

Richard Owen, one of the most renowned comparative anatomists and paleontologists of the day. After a year of study with Owen, Hitchcock returned to his alma mater to assume the position of hygiene director.[13]

Hitchcock's education abroad placed him within a generation of physicians who favored the "physiological method" of practice, which merged traditional therapeutics with the experimental science being conducted in the great European research laboratories.[14] Following in this vein, although Hitchcock did give medical treatment to students when needed, his primary goal was to prevent illness through regular exercise and training in hygienic manners of living. A key influence on Hitchcock's physical education program was Dio Lewis, whose physical education system particularly appealed to Hitchcock because it discarded the obsession with great muscular development that dominated physical culture prior to his arrival at Amherst. In the 1850s, Hitchcock recalled, traveling strongmen regularly offered displays of feats of strength, which "were then considered as indications of health, and held up to the students as the means for the true hygiene of life." In contrast, Hitchcock argued, "the most healthful and intellectual men" were well developed and of "excellent physical inheritance" but were not "*muscle* men." Although some ridiculed Lewis's exercises as suitable only for "girls and children," Hitchcock believed that thirty minutes of vigorous movement to a "polka or any lively music" was the best way to work the "whole man" while preventing "total exhaustion." Although he encouraged the talented few who "took naturally to heavy gymnastics" to cultivate their skills, he believed that light calisthenics were sufficient for the average students "who were sound in all four of their limbs and eyesight."[15]

Like his father, the younger Hitchcock saw the interconnectedness of spiritual and physical health. He therefore believed that exercise could prevent a variety of morally abhorrent behaviors, including drinking, carousing, and most importantly masturbation. According to Hitchcock, "The best medical authorities now regard regular and tolerably severe gymnastic exercise not only as a preventive of this vice, but as a curative agent where this habit has been already formed." For others, regular exercise provided a wholesome way to disperse "superfluous animal spirits" that built up during long hours of study and prayer.[16]

Hitchcock's work also was influenced by the "muscular Christianity" movement, which attempted to merge physical fitness and evangelical Protestantism. The term first appeared in the works of British author Thomas Hughes, whose *Tom Brown's Schooldays* (1857) and *Tom Brown at Oxford* (1860) promoted the virtues of "manliness, morality, health, and patriotism." Although the term *muscular Christianity* originated in Great Britain, it soon spread to other parts of the English-speaking world and took root in America, where the Second Great Awakening had created fertile ground for a movement that combined religious enlightenment and physical health. Hitchcock and other physical educators such as Lewis and Luther Gulick served as the leading U.S. apostles of muscular Christianity.[17]

Hitchcock found that his students were enthusiastic about the gymnasium and were generally respectful of his position as hygiene director. Hitchcock's popularity among the students may have resulted from his unusually high tolerance for the youthful exuberance of his charges as well as the relief the gymnasium provided from study and religious devotion. In 1866, Hitchcock reported to the trustees that the performance of students in his classes was "wonderful" during the most recent religious revival, as the "Gymnasium seemed to be at that time the safety valve for the escape of natural buoyancy of spirits that were pent up by the overpowering influence of religious impressions."[18]

To be sure, Hitchcock reported problems with students, especially during his early years. In a letter to Allen, Hitchcock wrote of the difficulty of creating a balance between order and recreation: "If I insist upon too much military authority," Hitchcock wrote, "I make the exercise heavy and deprive the young men of the means of completely throwing off all care and anxiety; and if I allow too much gaiety and natural exercise, I seem to have no authority or discipline."[19] Hitchcock also complained about students who wished to get out of physical education. Many of these excuses came "on account of direction or request from parents or physicians,—many of whom know nothing of our exercises except that they are styled 'gymnastics,' and hence infer that they are of the severer form of labor, such as formerly were always connected with gymnasia." Hitchcock observed that students themselves were less likely to ask for excuse. The few who did were "generally of the effeminate class, or the decidedly lazy ones."[20]

Hitchcock overcame attendance problems by rejecting "military authority" and allowing students more freedom than did faculty in other disciplines. According to Hitchcock, "College students will generally chafe under that rule which degrades them from the agents of free will and choice to a mere live machine, except when 'country calls.'" Hitchcock observed that another value of his program "has been its humanizing or leveling influence." Students who did not excel in the classroom could demonstrate their physical attainments or endurance in the gymnasium.

Regular physical exercise also undercut the elitism of the college's literary and social clubs, thereby preparing the college man "for the battle of life and the development of proper sympathies and self-denial." Above all, physical education mitigated some of the less wholesome aspects of male undergraduate life. According to Hitchcock, since the program had begun, the need for discipline decreased and the "drinking of intoxicating liquors, and the useless expenditure of money in style and show, which once were prevalent in college, are less during the few years past." As a result of his abandonment of "petty rules" and his respect for students' "control, government, and self-reliance," Hitchcock reported that students were less likely to shirk his courses than those offered by more rigid faculty members. Some students were so enthusiastic about gymnastics that they followed Hitchcock into careers in physical education.[21] Many students and alumni wrote fondly of their memories of "Old Doc." In a 1910 letter to Hitchcock, Levi H. Elwell, secretary of the Class of 1875, wrote of his and his classmates' "great debt of gratitude for all your loving kindness to us."[22]

The attempts to create a department of physical education and hygiene did not come without a struggle. From the outset, President Stearns and the trustees insisted that the department be put on the same status as other disciplines. This meant the director should be a "thoroughly trained physician" who was a full-time member of the faculty. Although faculty and other physicians in town agreed that the new physical director's work had definitely improved the health of the students, in an 1868 letter to Allen, Hitchcock wrote of his "embarrassment and difficulty of managing my department." Other faculty considered his work "experimental" and so did not give his department the same respect as more permanent subjects such as Latin, Greek, or natural history. Furthermore, there were no grades attached to physical education, as there were with other departments. Since "college rank is an engine of mighty power with students," Hitchcock lamented, "I am deprived of the most effective means of showing up my department on the college books." Finally, faculty attitudes toward exercise and physical training were "bordering on the edge of prize fighting, boat racing and horse training." Given all these factors, Hitchcock concluded, it was a wonder that students' attitude toward him was so cordial and respectful.[23]

In reply, Allen suggested that the best way to prove the worth of his work to other faculty was to explore the field of physical education in the same scientific spirit as had the elder Hitchcock: "The field is, in a great measure, new—untried—unexplored and experimental somewhat as the geological world was when your Father came on the stage," wrote Allen. "But, the field and its fruits, are far more important, as time will prove. In this, I am not mistaken. You will live to see it, though I may not."[24]

Allen was alluding to the emerging science of anthropometry, which gained ground in the 1860s after President Abraham Lincoln authorized the creation of the U.S. Sanitary Commission following catastrophic Union losses in the opening months of the Civil War. Although the new agency's main goals were improving medical care and disease prevention among the troops, the Sanitary Commission, along with private insurance companies interested in collecting actuarial data, funded a study to collect vital statistics on a million Union Army soldiers. In his final report to the Sanitary Commission, study director Benjamin A. Gould observed that the resulting data had broad implications not only for actuarial science but for medicine and public health as well.[25]

Allen's observations on the declining birthrate among the native-born, white inhabitants of New England extended these efforts to study the bodies of American men. Allen blamed the gradual extinction of the white race on the declining health and physical fitness of young men, particularly those in urban areas who worked in sedentary occupations.[26] Allen was also influenced by the work of Henry Pickering Bowditch, professor of physiology at Harvard Medical School who was responsible for conducting the first large-scale anthropometrical study of children, in the 1870s. Among Bowditch's more significant findings was the negative effect of factory labor on children's growth. Bowditch and his fellow physiologists also found that excessive "mental strain" could inhibit students' normal growth and development. The solution to these problems was the abolition of child labor and the promotion of physical exercise in the public schools.[27]

At Allen's urging, Hitchcock collected vital statistics on the students as a way of charting their progress in physical education classes as well as contributing to anthropometrical science. "If these statistics are continued for a series of years," Hitchcock noted in a report to the trustees in 1862, "they will be invaluable not only for Physiological Science, but also enable us to determine how far the Physical Department is of service to the College."[28]

In his compilation of twenty years of data on students' heights, weights, and other vital statistics, Hitchcock observed that the records of student health and illness compared "more favorably" to the records of other youth of the same age. Census returns and life insurance tables showed a decline in the "chance of life" among males aged fifteen to twenty-five in general. Hitchcock reported that Amherst medical records showed a variation from this statistic, as "sickness diminishes in our life here from 18 to 22 years of age." These facts led Hitchcock to conclude that college life was healthier than other occupations for young men.[29]

This emphasis on the health benefits of the college environment was meant to curb anxieties that the white, native-born, upper classes were dying out because of ill health, poor physical fitness, and lower birthrates than immigrants and African Americans. While many of these fears about race suicide focused on the health of college women, who married less often and then had fewer children than women who did not attend college, concerns about race suicide and racial degeneration were just as strong in discussions about the health of college men. Health experts warned the sedentary habits of an increasingly urbanized middle class were creating a generation of young men who were weak in both body and spirit. Noted neurologist George M. Beard claimed that excessive brain work at the expense of bodily development was the cause of a seeming "epidemic" of neurasthenia, characterized by nervous weakness and extreme physical fatigue. In comparison with the bodies of Native Americans, African Americans, and newly arrived immigrants, those of white native-born males seemed to be decidedly puny and weak.[30] Building manly bodies would become a bulwark against these threats to the white male body as well as the challenges posed by the independent, strong, and assertive "New Women" who were appearing on college campuses at this time.

Dudley Allen Sargent and the New College Man

Among the leaders in this effort to re-create the male college student body was Dr. Dudley Allen Sargent, who used his life story to illustrate the benefits of physical training for college men. Sargent was born in Belfast, Maine, in 1849. His father was a "strong and vigorous man" from whom Sargent "inherited a good physique, a strong will, a fondness for physical activity, and a love for good reading." From his mother, Sargent received a "nervous temperament," which "kept me ever at war with myself."[31]

Like many aspiring college men of his generation, Sargent supported his secondary and college education through a variety of manual jobs, including working in lumber camps, mills, and farms in and around his boyhood home. Among his more lucrative occupations was his work as a professional gymnast and circus performer, where he learned to develop and display a "powerful manhood." Yet Sargent "longed for something more permanent and stable than these vicarious positions. In other words," said Sargent, "I desired a profession." Sargent also hoped to dispel the "public prejudice" he met as both a performer and teacher of physical education. "The gymnasium was regarded in the same light as were billiard saloons and bowling alleys," Sargent recalled. "Whether this ill feeling was a survival of a Puritanical spirit that tended to stamp out all manifestations of life and joyousness, or whether its cause lay in the custom of the German turners in performing in cheap recreation halls and saloons, I cannot say."[32]

In fall of 1869, Sargent entered Bowdoin College, supporting himself by working as the director of the college's gymnasium. Like his counterparts at other institutions, Sargent found no difficulty in getting naturally athletic students, many of whom worked on farms, factories, and lumber camps to earn their tuition, to take an interest in exercise. However, his major challenge was persuading men "who had mental ability, but who were physically weak" to attend the gymnasium. These students, Sargent observed, were unlikely to take gymnastic exercises seriously unless an edict came from the faculty and administration. Like Hitchcock, Sargent collected data to demonstrate the effectiveness of his exercise program. By 1872, he had convinced the faculty to require mandatory attendance at the gymnasium five days per week. As a result of his work, Sargent reported in 1874, the "average health of the students has vastly improved, and many people commented upon the high tone of the college morals."[33]

Sargent eventually realized that if his physical education work was to gain scientific legitimacy, he needed further training in science and medicine. After graduating from Bowdoin, he entered Yale Medical College in 1875. While at Yale, Sargent worked on devising his system of exercise and physical development. When he received his M.D. in 1878, Sargent applied to almost a dozen college presidents, offering to introduce his new system to their institutions. Much to his dismay, Sargent found that no one was interested in his idea of creating a department of physical training that would merge physiology, hygiene instruction, psychology, sociology, and ethics. Sargent concluded, "My fight was no longer with the boys, but with those higher up."[34]

Sargent then left New Haven to set up a hygienic institute in New York City. Both his family and his college friends scoffed at his work. Sargent's associates at Yale Medical School saw this as a "radical departure" from his training in regular medicine, believing he was "entering upon a career of medical quackery." His work attracted the attention of Alexander Agassiz, son of acclaimed Harvard zoologist Louis Agassiz and curator of the natural history museum at Harvard. Sargent also came in contact with Harvard alumnus and star athlete William Blaikie, a prominent New York lawyer, who enthusiastically endorsed the Sargent system in his best-selling book, *How to Get Strong and How to Stay So*.[35]

Both Agassiz and Blaikie were instrumental in securing Sargent's appointment at Harvard, where President Eliot agreed that enhancing the prominence of physical education in the curriculum would further ensure the bodily superiority of Harvard undergraduates. Following the Amherst model, Eliot put physical education on an equal standing with other academic departments. Physical education courses were not mandatory, however. Although Sargent offered physical education to all students who wished to take it, he found that the sickliest and weakest students were the least likely to use the gymnasium. Sargent also encountered serious opposition from the trustees and faculty members, many of whom believed that "physical training was not a profession worthy of the efforts of an educated man."[36]

Nevertheless, the establishment of a gymnasium at Harvard attracted the attention of other colleges and universities, which sought to emulate Sargent's work. In response, Sargent set up a summer school of physical education to train men for similar programs at other men's colleges, coeducational institutions, and boys' schools. The spread of the Sargent system to other institutions caused many of Sargent's colleagues "who had looked upon the profession as a hobby of cranks and half-educated folk" to change their attitude toward the new science of physical fitness.[37] To Sargent, physical education appeared to be on its way to becoming a legitimate academic discipline.

A Scientific Spirit of Manly Excellence

Among Sargent's more notable protégés was R. Tait McKenzie at the University of Pennsylvania. McKenzie attended the Harvard summer school and during the 1890s compiled Sargent's data to create statues of "typical" American college men and women from measurements collected during mandatory physical examinations at elite men's and women's colleges. Prominently displayed in the Anthropology Building at the 1893 Chicago World's Columbian Exposition, these statues illustrated the bodily superiority of college men and women compared to the "barbaric" bodies of Native Americans, African Americans, and "foreign races" exhibited in the fair's Midway attractions.[38]

At the same time, McKenzie warned, modern civilization was having a negative impact on the physiques of American youth. He observed, "American youth does not show up so badly" but were considerably thinner and less muscled than the broad-shouldered, heavy-set "Herculean" types of ancient Greece. Although McKenzie acknowledged that a certain degree of slenderness and delicacy of figure was the sign of a "refined and highly civilized race," he also warned that too much "softness of form" in men was a sign of racial degeneracy.[39] According to McKenzie, evidence of impending race suicide was especially apparent in city dwellers like those who attended the University of Pennsylvania: "The segregation of masses of people limits the amount of space and air for each," McKenzie wrote, "and the necessity of further economizing energy by the use of machinery reduces muscular activity to a minimum."[40] Although the physical problems caused by urban living could be detected in all social classes, McKenzie found them especially apparent in the most civilized members of society, leading to a host of diseases and defects caused by lack of regular muscular activity. Men who attended college were especially at risk, as the stress and strain of college education was "frequently stamped on the physique of the matriculant."[41]

McKenzie believed the best way to counteract this trend was for men's colleges to support physical education as fully as they did other academic programs. Many campuses offered physical education to all students who wished to take it, but if these classes were not mandatory, physical educators found that the ones who most needed exercise were also the most likely to avoid it. When Penn first started its program in physical education in 1885, students did not have to take physical education classes and were more inclined to engage in athletics and interclass fights than to visit the gymnasium. A desire to redirect students' passion for games, fights, and class rivalries into more acceptable channels led the university to build Franklin Field, complete construction of Weightman Gymnasium, and appoint McKenzie to supervise the physical education department. Unlike previous physical education directors, McKenzie's position was full time, and he received full faculty status. The trustees also approved the most stringent physical education requirement of any university in the country at that time. All students received a physical examination upon entrance to the university, a practice that had become common at many institutions of higher education by the turn of the century. Students also had to take a minimum of two physical education classes per week for all four years at the university, whereas most colleges only required a year of physical education or had no such requirements at all. Students at the University of Pennsylvania received the same academic credit for physical education as for other subjects but also received the same penalties as for other required courses. Students could not graduate unless they fulfilled the physical education requirement, and they were not allowed to sit for final examinations if they had skipped physical education classes during the preceding semester.[42]

Students had other ideas. According to McKenzie, although some students welcomed the opportunity to improve their bodies for academic credit, others objected to the intrusion on their time, staging a protest at which they burned McKenzie in effigy. McKenzie also continually clashed with the Athletic Association and the coaches over whether athletes could be excused from the physical education requirement and whether McKenzie should have final say over who was fit for competition. The faculty also resisted the physical education requirements. McKenzie observed that many professors viewed physical education "as a sort of bastard child left on their doorstep, diverting the time and nourishment destined only for legitimately begotten members of the academic faculty."[43]

To establish academic legitimacy, McKenzie and others in the emerging field of physical education strove to demonstrate the physiological benefits of exercise and thereby set their discipline on firm scientific footing. Gymnasia became laboratories aimed at establishing physical education as a bona fide science. The professional organization for physical educators, the American Association for the Advancement of Physical Education, established in 1885, modeled its title after the American Association for the Advancement of Science. Like Hitchcock, many of the leaders in the field were trained in medicine, they founded the association to establish "rational, scientific study" of the effects of exercise on mind and body.[44]

Among the most illustrious members of the Association for the Advancement of Physical Education was Edward M. Hartwell, a former student of Hitchcock. After graduating from Amherst, Hartwell received a medical degree from Cincinnati Miami Medical College and a doctorate in biology from Johns Hopkins University, which employed him as an instructor in physical culture and director of the gymnasium from 1882 to 1890. Hartwell's appointment constituted part of Hopkins president Daniel Coit Gilman's effort to build the scientific reputation of the new institution while paying due attention to the "physical side" of the student body. To this end, he wanted someone who was thoroughly trained in both biological science and medicine.[45] Hartwell declared in an 1885 report on the status of physical training in American colleges that the "modern" place of physical training "is the child of the scientific spirit embodied in the new physiology and the new psychology" espoused by leading scientists of the day. This new "scientific spirit" presented not only a new model for physical education but also a new ideal of "manly excellence" that should "determine all our schemes and endeavors for the nurture and training of youth." Hartwell claimed that the product of a liberal education should be a man who is "no stunted ascetic" but "is full of life and fire, but whose passions are trained to come to heel by a vigorous will, the servant of tender conscience; who has learned to love all beauty, whether of nature or of art, to hate all vileness, and to respect others as himself." Because physical education was at its base a medical science, Hartwell argued, control of college gymnasia should be taken "out of the hands of ignorant and low-toned trainers and athletes" and placed "into the hands of educated medical men" trained in regular medicine. According to Hartwell, "The director of a college gymnasium should possess sufficient academic and professional training to entitle him to a place in the Faculty, and to ensure him the respect of his colleagues." He should be "a friendly medical, or rather hygienic, adviser of young men to their habits of study, exercise, and recreation." Above all, the gymnasium director, not the coaches, should judge whether a young man was fit to engage in athletic contests and exhibitions.[46] These claims to expert authority over the male student body would not go unchallenged.

Civilized Yet Manly

College men did not always willingly accept the notion that their bodies needed restructuring. The determination of the young Theodore Roosevelt to overcome his childhood asthma and "puny sickly body" is a prime example of how male undergraduates' "body projects" defied those of medical authorities.[47] The wealth and social prominence of Roosevelt's family ensured young Teddy's admission to Harvard, but after a physical examination, Sargent informed Roosevelt that his asthma and heart problems indicated that he should refrain from physical exertion of any kind. Roosevelt refused to follow this advice and went on to become a star athlete at Harvard as well as a proponent of how the "strenuous life" could help anyone overcome physical or mental adversity.[48]

Of course, a desire to protect professional turf played some role in physical educators' outcry against athletics, since these programs were controlled largely by alumni and students. However, physical education directors had legitimate complaints based on the best scientific evidence of the day. Like college administrators and faculty, physical educators objected to what they considered the rampant dishonesty, violence, and commercialism of college sports. Early athletic contests were also dangerous: it was not unusual for a college to list a dozen or more deaths and/or serious injuries from athletic competitions throughout the year. Physical educators were also concerned about a condition called "athlete's heart." Autopsies showed that the hearts of former athletes were enlarged, a condition attributed to the excessive stress of college sports.[49] Most importantly, physical educators opposed the elitism inherent in most college athletic programs. They argued that rather than funding athletic programs that served only a small number of students, colleges should support programs that benefited all students equally. Although McKenzie acknowledged that physical education departments should make provisions for the "supernormal" athletes as well as for "subnormal" students with physical defects, the main goal of such programs should be to serve the "average man" who "has neither the desire nor the ability to represent his university upon the track or field, but who wishes to be at his highest point of physical vigor throughout his college course." Only by supporting "exercise for all" could colleges and universities cultivate the qualities by which "civilized man has asserted and maintained his superiority over more primitive races."[50]

Of course, in this context, the term *civilized man* referred to the white, native-born, middle-class men who comprised the majority of male collegians in the late nineteenth century. Yet colleges for black men adopted similar ideas about the relationship between physical fitness and manhood. Among the more prominent colleges for black men at this time were Fisk University in Nashville and Howard University in Washington, D.C. Although both offered vocational training as a way for poorer students to earn money for tuition and room and board (as well as provide the institutions with cheap labor), these universities also believed liberal education and cultivation of good moral character to be essential to their missions. Like white colleges and universities, Fisk and Howard were concerned with developing a "Christian manhood" that made moral education indispensable "for instilling in black men the qualities and traits that were necessary for attaining Victorian manliness." As at white institutions, a key component of moral education was mandatory physical education, which would help young black men develop racially fit bodies. Yet regulating black male student behavior was even more critical than at white institutions, since rules were aimed at counteracting racist stereotypes about black male sexuality. To further enhance the students' moral education, both Fisk and Howard imposed strict parietal rules on their students. At Howard, student life resembled that at a military camp: male students woke to reveille; wore uniforms; marched to and from classes, meals, and religious services; attended daily military drills; and ended the day with mandatory lights out. Fisk also closely regulated the lives of students, but regulations were modeled after the black middle-class family. Students and faculty lived in the same residence halls and ate together in a common dining room, traditions meant to make campus life resemble that of respectable homes.[51]

These developments at elite black colleges provided a striking contrast to the educational environment for white college men. By the late nineteenth century, most custodial policies for male students had been abolished, if they had ever existed. This trend resulted largely from mid-nineteenth-century student riots during which many white male students rebelled against what they considered outmoded school policies. Students complained about unfair tutors, bad food, poorly lit and dirty accommodations, and above all the monastic social rules imposed by the strict overseers. Some even went to further extremes and rioted against, beat, horsewhipped, or stoned professors and presidents who did not acquiesce to their demands.[52]

Many college administrators also believed that white men did not need the same supervision as women because they were men, not boys. This became especially true after the Civil War, when the average age of male students increased to eighteen. According to renowned neurologist S. Weir Mitchell, male students of eighteen or nineteen were well beyond the "age of development." They therefore had "no physiological need" for the close supervision imposed on female students or young boys.[53]

Harvard's Eliot likewise argued that students did not need the parietal rules imposed on boys precisely because they were men or at least nearly so: the average age of Harvard students in the 1860s was over eighteen, significantly older than students a century earlier. Eliot hoped that removing parietal regulations would eliminate the "schoolboy spirit" that characterized antebellum men's colleges. As Eliot put it, "The refining influences of liberal study and good companionship, rather than . . . strictness of regulation" would encourage good behavior among the students.[54]

Colleges with fewer financial resources than those in the Ivy League simply could not afford to provide more than the most minimal accommodations for their students.[55] In addition, many did not believe supervision of male students to be part of their educational missions. Instead, many college presidents and administrators believed that the sole purpose of a university was teaching and research. American land-grant universities emulated those in Germany, which did not regulate students' extracurricular activities. American university leaders, therefore, believed that their male students should be left to fend for themselves as well.[56]

Hitchcock was the first to suggest that this situation was unacceptable, arguing that the success of Mount Holyoke and other colleges in protecting female student health resulted from the fact that disease prevention did not end at the gymnasium door. Drawing on the model provided by the U.S. Sanitary Commission during the war, Hitchcock argued that colleges should provide the same attention to sanitary conditions on and around campus as did military organizations.[57] According to Hitchcock, the "life of the student is as healthful as are the lives of other occupations, if not more so," but he also observed that the "student in the ordinary boarding-house or college dormitory is certainly no better cared for than are most young men of the same age of the mercantile and many of the artisan class." Nor was there any "evidence that the student, with his inheritance and early environment, starts in life any better 'selected' than do his play-mates who enter the store, machine-shop, or the farm."[58] In a report to the American Public Health Association in 1878, Hitchcock observed that it was a miracle that Amherst students escaped relatively unscathed during a major epidemic of typhoid fever in Massachusetts the preceding year. According to board of health statistics, the number of "deaths of males from typhoid fever were 742, while those of females were but 663. Still further, 42 per cent of the deaths from this same cause were between the ages of 15 and 30 years (Amherst students average 21 years and 2 months)." Hitchcock added that 44 percent of these deaths occurred during the first three months of the fall term. Given this data, "combined with the fact that students are not at home, and are at the 'daring and inconsiderate' age," Hitchcock concluded, it was a wonder more cases of typhoid had not occurred among the student body.[59] Although student health remained good, Hitchcock warned that the college might not always be so fortunate since the campus lacked the "system of and discipline of the sanitary organization in our army and navy."[60]

By the early 1900s, new discoveries in bacteriology and major epidemics of contagious diseases in college towns increasingly demonstrated that more aggressive measures needed to be taken to not only build the bodies of young white men but also protect them from environmental dangers both on and off campus.

CHAPTER 3

Sending Their Sons into Danger

In 1903, the city of Ithaca, New York, was hit by a devastating epidemic of typhoid fever. Among the city population as a whole, which numbered 15,800 permanent residents and students, 1,350 cases of typhoid occurred, resulting in 82 deaths. Cornell University students were hit especially hard by the epidemic, partly because adolescents and young adults were the most vulnerable age groups for this disease. By the time the epidemic ended in the fall, 291 students had contracted typhoid fever, with 29 deaths.[1]

Ithaca was not the first college town to experience an epidemic of this magnitude, nor would it be the last. What made the event newsworthy was how sharply it contrasted with larger trends in public health and preventive medicine. As early as the 1860s, many scientists and members of the lay public strongly suspected that careless methods of sewage disposal and an unsanitary environment were among the major causes of many infectious diseases. According to this zymotic theory of contagion first postulated by the German chemist Justus von Leibig, disease resulted from noxious odors emitted from rotting or fermenting matter. This theory appeared to be confirmed by surveys conducted by the U.S. Sanitary Commission and state and local health officials that demonstrated a strong correlation between "filth" in the environment and epidemic diseases such as cholera and typhoid fever. Advice literature from this period popularized the notion "dirt equals disease" and instructed homemakers on how to rid their houses of all sources of filth and foul air.[2] In Massachusetts, such findings were one of the major justifications for the creation of the board of health in 1869, the nation's first state public health agency. In the 1870s, the board gained increasing authority to regulate pollution by slaughterhouses, tanneries, factories, and other "public nuisances." Yet individual towns and cities still retained a large degree of individual autonomy from state regulation. Consequently, sanitary conditions varied greatly throughout the Commonwealth.[3]

During the 1880s, bacteriologists demonstrated that microorganisms caused diseases such as cholera and typhoid fever. Even apparently clean and odor-free water, food, and homes could harbor these bacteria. This gave public health experts the ability to more precisely trace sources of epidemics to water and food supplies that had been contaminated by waste from those infected with the disease. These discoveries led to calls for reforms in waste management and sanitary engineering. By the early twentieth century, a number of major cities, including New York and Philadelphia, had installed sewers, waste treatment plants, and water filtration systems to prevent the spread of typhoid fever, cholera, dysentery, and other waterborne infectious diseases.[4]

Thus, many observers familiar with the public health advances of the early-twentieth-century United States saw the epidemic in Ithaca as an easily foreseeable and preventable tragedy. Newspapers and magazines around the country accused the city and university of gross ignorance and neglect of even the most rudimentary methods of preventive medicine. In the words of *McClure's*, one of the leading muckraking periodicals of the era, the Ithaca epidemic exemplified "unprogressiveness in matters of public health which so strangely contrasts with the forwarding American spirit" of the early twentieth century.[5]

This outcry underestimated the degree to which popular resistance to public health reform persisted well after scientific discoveries demonstrated the importance of preventive measures such as water filtration and mandatory vaccination. Despite reformers' message that "public health was purchasable," American taxpayers often hesitated to fund such efforts, especially when they benefited "social undesirables" such as African Americans, Native Americans, and the immigrant poor. Moreover, the notion that the state had a responsibility to protect the health of its citizens conflicted with American values of individualism, self-reliance, and limited government. Therefore, while public health reforms were becoming increasingly common in Europe, a public health infrastructure was slower to develop in the United States and greatly depended on local circumstances. In general, many middle-class Americans preferred to focus on improving sanitary conditions in their homes than on calling for community reforms. Drawing on popular domestic hygiene literature of the day, those who could afford to do so installed indoor plumbing fixtures, sewer traps, and other home improvements geared at creating a sanitary household environment. Much like today, those who suspected contamination of public water supplies dug their own private wells or relied on bottled springwater imported from popular spa areas such as Saratoga Springs.[6]

This chapter will explore how notions of gender and race shaped the way campuses responded to threats of epidemics and contagious disease. As chapter 1 demonstrated, warnings about the allegedly harmful affects of higher education on the health of young women led women's colleges and coeducational institutions to require women to live on campus, where their moral and physical well-being could be closely monitored. Black colleges for both men and women also imposed strict regulations on their students as a means of counteracting racist stereotypes depicting blacks as a "degenerate" and disease-prone race.

During most of the nineteenth century, officials were reluctant to assume the same responsibility for white male students in loco parentis, instead allowing them to reside wherever they chose. This did not mean that colleges and universities completely ignored bad personal habits. In fact, many institutions explicitly banned drinking, gambling, profanity, and other unacceptable forms of behavior. Cornell, for example, regularly expelled students for drunkenness and disorderly conduct. Attempts to enforce campus rules of conduct encountered difficulty, however, because most men did not reside on campus. In fact, some college and university administrators believed that housing male students together contributed to their unruly behavior. Cornell's first president, Andrew Dickson White, agreed to house a limited number of male students on campus yet was "opposed, on principle, to dormitories for men." White insisted that "professors should not have to play the part of spies and policemen" for youthful exuberance. Remembering the turbulence in the residence halls of his undergraduate and graduate school days, White insisted that male students were best off under the care of Ithaca's "high-minded landladies" who ran boardinghouses.[7]

Wealthier students at both private and public institutions made up for these deficiencies in campus offerings by creating fraternities, dining clubs, and secret societies. However, fraternities did not necessarily provide a healthier alternative to the boardinghouses: like their modern-day counterparts, turn-of-the-century fraternities condoned smoking, drinking, gambling, and other activities that at best diverted students from the educational mission of the university and at worst posed serious risks to their health. The fraternity buildings themselves were also hazardous: a number of fraternities were destroyed by fire during the 1890s and early 1900s, and four students died in a fire at Cornell's Chi Psi fraternity in 1906.[8] The father of one of the men who died wrote that "University authorities would do well" to inspect other fraternities and boardinghouses occupied by Cornell students "to protect the University from accusations and implications which another fire of this kind would bring forth." If house owners and fraternities did not cooperate, then university authorities should make sure "that ample protection is provided everywhere."[9]

Moreover, these options were available only to those who had the economic status or social connections to be accepted into these elite organizations. At public institutions, some students solved the housing problem by commuting from family homes or living with relatives near campus. By the 1880s, it became common for families with college-age sons and daughters to move to growing "gown towns" like Bloomington, Indiana, and Ann Arbor, Michigan, so that their children could attend college while living at home. These families frequently would take in boarders and remain in town after their children graduated, thereby providing accommodations for future generations of students. Junior faculty would often supplement their meager salaries by taking in boarders as well. College officials believed that these "family-run" establishments were "wholesome and conducive to university life" by providing the comforts and supervision that students would receive in their own homes. But "proper" families never had enough rooms to meet the demand. At the same time, new boarding establishments run by individuals interested mainly in earning a profit rather than providing surrogate homes became more numerous.[10]

This gender disparity in housing and student supervision became increasingly intolerable to parents of college men. In the words of one mother who wrote to Cornell president Jacob Gould Schurman following the 1903 typhoid epidemic, "How long are parents going to send their sons into such danger? . . . [M]ust we transfer our son to some other college where the health of the students is of first consideration?"[11] By the early twentieth century, many other parents of college men had adopted similar expectations that colleges would replicate the standards of hygiene and behavioral oversight adopted by most middle-class homes. These new views prompted colleges and universities to take a more proactive approach to protecting male student health from environmental hazards both on and off campus.

Protecting Student Bodies in "Filthy-delphia"

During the late nineteenth century, the city of Philadelphia received a major blow to its former glory as the City of Brotherly Love. Reports about corruption in city government, crowded immigrant tenements, epidemics of infectious diseases, and inadequate control of public health earned the city the moniker Filthy-delphia. In the words of the noted journalist and reformer Lincoln Steffens, Philadelphia was a "disgrace" not only to itself and Pennsylvania "but to the United States and American character."[12] The University of Pennsylvania's administrators were embarrassed to discover that many trustees and alumni preferred to send their sons to rural colleges because parents presumed the absence of the physical dangers of the city would promote good physical and moral health.[13]

Concerns about the physical and moral quality of the neighborhood surrounding the University of Pennsylvania prompted a move during the 1870s from Ninth Street to a new campus in West Philadelphia. Considered a "genteel" neighborhood in the early nineteenth century, the area around Washington Square had become increasingly run-down after the Civil War as wealthier families abandoned the area for more fashionable quarters, leaving recent immigrants and decrepit student boardinghouses. In 1870, worried that the Ninth Street neighborhood was "vile" and "growing viler every day," university officials purchased ten acres of farmland west of the Schuylkill River in what was then semirural West Philadelphia. Administrators believed that this location was "ideally situated for a community requiring academic quiet and comparative isolation."[14]

The new campus initially included no dormitories, since the university wanted to avoid the expense and inconvenience of supervising young men. Furthermore, administrators reasoned that most students "came decorously every morning from their parents' homes on Walnut Street or from far-off Germantown, and were safely home by candlelight." The occasional out-of-state student was there "only because he had friends in Philadelphia, with whom he could find a safe and real home."[15]

However, changes in the university's institutional mission led administrators to begin reconsidering this policy during the 1880s and 1890s. At this time, Penn attempted to recruit students from outside of Philadelphia and its suburbs as part of a larger effort to make the university a nationally respected institution.[16] To this end, the university added eight new academic programs and expanded its course offerings to attract students from around the country. Convincing students from "away" to attend the University of Pennsylvania also meant assuring parents who lived long distances from campus that their sons were adequately protected from physical and moral harm. According to Provost Charles Custis Harrison, the time spent in college constituted a "formative epoch" in a young man's life, and a university had the duty to provide "all that life at that age requires (physically, socially, intellectually, morally and religiously)." The university could not completely meet students' needs, Harrison argued, until all students could find a "proper home which is in and of the university," with "careful provision for all the twenty-four hours of the students' daily life."[17] During the early 1890s, administrators discovered that one thousand students, or half of the entire student body, lived near the university in boardinghouses and fraternities, where they lacked any kind of supervision. Although the majority of students at this time came from wealthy families, a significant number of students had limited incomes that forced them to live under hazardous and unhealthy conditions.[18]

This great disparity between wealthy and low-income students was especially disturbing because Penn prided itself on its ability to attract a socioeconomically diverse cross-section of students from city and suburb. Since its inception, the university had projected an image of inclusiveness that supposedly welcomed students from every quarter. Reality frequently fell short of this image, since the university was priced beyond the reach of many immigrants and minorities. Temple College of Philadelphia, founded in 1888, was the city's true "workingman's college." The University of Pennsylvania did become more socioeconomically diverse after the Civil War, mainly because the sons of Philadelphia's wealthiest families favored more prestigious institutions located in pristine, immigrant-free areas. By the turn of the century, University of Pennsylvania students from the elite neighborhood around Rittenhouse Square were outnumbered almost four to one by those from the less fashionable but still prosperous wards in North, Northwest, and West Philadelphia. In addition, a small but significant number of students, 12 percent, came from poorer southern wards, Kensington, and the Northeast.[19] Therefore, there is some truth to the University of Pennsylvania's claim that it promoted a "democracy of the streetcar," since it was significantly more socioeconomically diverse than other elite men's colleges. One report from the turn of the century contrasted the luxurious living conditions of the "well set up and well-groomed young men" who resided in fraternities and plush apartments near the university with the "pale-faced, stoop-shouldered young men who snatch ravenously at a scrap of learning and hurry away with it to unknown parts of the city." Race was another matter, however; like other members of the Ivy League, Penn openly discriminated against Jewish and African

American applicants, limiting admissions to a few token members of these minorities.[20]

To preserve its self-image as a democratic institution, the University of Pennsylvania had to equalize student living conditions. To solve this problem, the administration looked to the residential colleges of Oxford and Cambridge for inspiration. These institutions had long traditions of using architecture to shape the lives of their students, but they also had reputations for social elitism. The Gothic architecture favored by proponents of the Oxbridge movement in American colleges and universities symbolized a larger movement to reassert Anglo-Saxon racial superiority in a rapidly changing social order.[21]

Trustees at the University of Pennsylvania were likewise concerned that their school was "marked by a singular deficiency in its instrumentalities for promoting religious and moral life." In 1893, the trustees approved a plan to construct Houston Hall, the first student union in the country, which was modeled after the gothic architecture of Oxford and Cambridge.[22] At the same time, the trustees announced plans for student dormitories, construction of which began in 1895. Unlike other elite universities at this time, the University of Pennsylvania lacked the financial resources to build dormitories for all of its students. Therefore, the university could not fulfill its hope of providing all students with affordable housing. Instead, administrators relied on the city's Progressive Era sanitary improvements, including the latest methods of sewage disposal, street cleaning, and water filtration.[23]

The Agrarian Myth and Public Health in Ithaca

In small college towns such as Ithaca, an agrarian myth of a healthful, self-reliant community made both town and gown reluctant to invest in many of the major health reforms that had already occurred in larger metropolitan areas such as Philadelphia. Parents, students, college officials, and residents alike believed that rural college towns were free from the massive public health problems that plagued most large cities by the middle of the nineteenth century. Furthermore, rural campuses were believed to be insulated from such evil temptations of the city as prostitution, gambling, drinking, and other vices. Fears about the impact of immigration added fuel to this image of agrarian purity, as concerns about the allegedly filthy habits of recent immigrants led many white, native-born parents to prefer rural colleges where their children would not have to mingle with "dirty foreigners."[24]

In Ithaca, the physical beauty and apparent healthfulness of the surrounding countryside caused many residents to believe their community was free from the disease and physical corruption that affected New York, Philadelphia, and other large urban centers. This image of Ithaca as a disease-free paradise may have been true in its early years, when the city's population was small. However, during the decades following the founding of Cornell University in 1868, Ithaca experienced a period of tremendous growth. The university's need for classrooms and faculty living quarters drew builders, merchants, and professionals to the village. University students often settled in town after graduation since they considered Ithaca an ideal place to live and raise a family. Between 1865 and 1903, the city's population more than doubled. Although Ithaca's size paled in comparison to the large industrial cities of the Northeast, by the early 1900s, Ithaca was no longer a little country town.[25]

Ithaca was also becoming more ethnically diverse, as foreign-born itinerant laborers and their families came to work in various construction and service jobs. These new arrivals resided primarily in a neighborhood known by local residents as the Silent City or the Rhine, which ran along the Cascadilla Creek Inlet in the southwestern portion of the city. Since few homes in this area had indoor plumbing, the inlet served as an open sewer for the neighborhood as well as a dumping ground for liquid and solid waste from the rest of the city. Cornell University and the wealthier neighborhoods atop East Hill pumped their sewage directly into Silent City's water source. During rainstorms and ice thaws, effluvia from hilltop neighborhoods flowed directly into the inlet, making the water unsafe for human consumption and leading to a high incidence of waterborne diseases among the neighborhood's inhabitants.[26]

Since typhoid fever and other filth diseases appeared to affect only the most wretched of the city's residents, Ithaca's middle class hesitated to pay the extra taxes needed for municipal improvements. Another obstacle to public health reform was the long-standing conflict between the city and the university. Although some Ithacans welcomed students and faculty as a source of business and expertise, others were suspicious of the "new ideas, new longings, and new fears" fostered by this influx of "rowdy students and cosmopolitan professors."[27] In particular, Cornell scientists' calls for public health reforms clashed with residents' perceptions about the supposed healthfulness of the city.

Even if municipal public health reforms within the city limits had succeeded, many Ithaca residents would still have been powerless to control the quality of the city water supply, which came from two separate sources running through hamlets and villages outside of Ithaca. The drainage area of the larger source, Six Mile Creek, had a 1903 population of about 2,144, of whom 812 lived in villages bordering the creek. Drainage from area cesspools, privies, and barnyards flowed directly into the creek and its tributaries. Residents who lived along the watershed dumped their trash directly onto the banks of the creek. There was no system of purifying the water, except for a primitive crib filter that sifted out pebbles and other large objects. The second water supply was Buttermilk Creek, which duplicated on a smaller scale the sanitary conditions of Six Mile Creek. During periods of dry weather, vast quantities of refuse of all descriptions (including manure and dead animals) accumulated on the banks of the creeks and their tributaries, and heavy rains and thaws scoured this garbage down into the water supply. The conditions along these watersheds therefore made it very easy for waterborne diseases such as typhoid to enter the city's water supply.[28]

Although the solutions to Ithaca's water problems were obvious to scientific experts from Cornell University and the Ithaca Board of Health, neither institution had control over the towns and villages that bordered the city water supply. Consequently, these officials could not order residents of these areas to remove outhouses, cesspools, manure piles, and other public health nuisances that threatened Ithaca's water supply.[29]

Many Ithacans complained about the taste and smell of city water, instead relying on water from private wells or artesian water brought to the city by vendors. For at least two years prior to the epidemic, chemical and bacteriological examinations of the city water made by Professor Emile Chamot of the Cornell Department of Chemistry and Professor V. A. Moore of the Department of Bacteriology and published in the daily papers warned Ithacans that city water was unfit for drinking in the raw state, especially after heavy rains and spring flooding. Visitors to the city were warned about "Ithaca fever" or "Six Mile Colitis," said to be caused by the city's water supply. Newcomers to Ithaca were especially prone to these maladies. People under twenty-five years of age were more vulnerable than any other age group. At least 10 to 15 percent of each entering class at Cornell University contracted "freshman diarrhea" because of the water supply. During the five years prior to the epidemic, some cases of "Ithaca fever" had been treated at the student infirmary each year. In the winter of 1900–1901, between 40 and 50 of these student cases occurred, and in 1901–2, the number increased to around 150. In addition, some cases of typhoid were present in the city hospital and the student infirmary each year. For example, in the fall of 1902, the city hospital treated 14 cases of typhoid assumed to have originated from the city water supply.[30]

Popular distrust of the water supply was compounded by the fact that the city's water company was privately owned. Like other late-nineteenth-century Americans, Ithaca residents became increasingly suspicious of privately owned big businesses that monopolized public utilities.[31] The Treman family established the Ithaca Water Works Company in 1872. Two years earlier, the majority of Ithaca taxpayers had voted against a proposal that the village raise one hundred thousand dollars in taxes to construct a waterworks to be owned and operated by the village. In 1873, a year after the Treman brothers began construction of their waterworks, the trustees of the village again proposed to buy the rights and franchises of the Ithaca Water Works Company, and again they were defeated. Despite the fact that many Ithacans and Cornell officials felt that it was in Ithaca's best interest to have municipal control over the source "of either the good or ill health of the city," special elections for municipal ownership were defeated twice more in 1900 and 1902.[32]

Hostility toward the privately owned water company, combined with apathy regarding the plight of the city's less fortunate residents, led many Ithaca taxpayers to focus on keeping infection at bay in their homes. Drawing on popular domestic hygiene literature of the day, middle-class Ithacans installed indoor plumbing fixtures, sewer traps, and other home improvements geared at creating a sanitary, germ-free household environment.[33] Those who could afford to do so constructed their own wells for drinking water rather than relying on the Ithaca Water Works Company. The wealthiest families attempted to avoid the problem of contamination altogether by purchasing bottled springwater from private vendors, but studies conducted during the epidemic indicated that water sellers were not always reliable, and these sources too could be tainted.[34]

Given what was known about the condition of the city water supply, it is not surprising that Ithaca residents preferred private solutions to public health problems. Unfortunately, the private wells used by approximately one-third of the city's residents were also a potential source of danger. A number of them were too shallow to avoid receiving drainage from nearby cesspools, outhouses, and sewer lines. During the 1903 typhoid epidemic, the board of health discovered that more than 30 percent of the city's thirteen hundred–plus private wells were unfit for drinking purposes.[35] More importantly, not everyone in the city had the financial resources to invest in private solutions to public health dangers. The Rhiners were the most likely to contract waterborne infectious diseases because of their wretched living conditions and their reliance on water from the polluted Cascadilla Creek Inlet.

Another obstacle to public health reform was the long-standing conflict between Ithaca residents and members of the university community that existed since Cornell opened its doors. Cornell scientists' calls for public health reforms clashed with residents' perceptions about the supposed healthfulness of the city, and local citizens became extremely upset at the suggestion that their fair city needed sanitary improvements. Tensions between town and gown were so great the university could not even control the sanitary condition of its own water supply. The Cornell campus received its water from a different source than did the city—Fall Creek—but the sanitary condition of this supply were no better than Six Mile and Buttermilk Creeks. As early as 1880, Cornell president Andrew Dickson White suspected that the water from Fall Creek was responsible for illnesses among students and faculty members. White asked Professors A. A. Breneman and George C. Caldwell of the Department of Chemistry and Dr. James Law of the veterinary college to survey the conditions along Fall Creek. Breneman reported extremely hazardous systems of sewage and waste disposal bordering the creek, causing an uproar among the residents along Fall Creek. Most of them received their water from private wells and thus saw no reason to cooperate with the university's request to clean up the Fall Creek watershed. Instead, they called for Breneman's firing. White refused, stating that he would rather "see the whole of the University tumbled into Cayuga Lake" than dismiss the young man for "attempting to call the people to a sense of their duty to themselves, their children, and the University." Nevertheless, community pressure forced Breneman to seek his fortune elsewhere, and the university continued to be stymied in its attempts to clean up the campus water supply.[36]

In 1902, things had become so grave that Cornell officials enlisted the New York State commissioner of health, Dr. Daniel Lewis, to help regulate the sanitary conditions of the university water supply. Lewis drew up a list of rules and regulations prohibiting inhabitants along Fall Creek and its tributaries from depositing any sort of refuse or excrement in the creeks and from building any privies, cesspools, or sewers along Fall Creek or its tributaries.[37] These regulations were not widely observed, however. During the 1903 epidemic, for example, Cornell scientists and state health officials found numerous violations of state sanitary regulations as well as a high concentration of intestinal bacteria in the Fall Creek water supply. Because women students were required to live in the Sage College dormitory, university officials could compensate for the poor quality of water from Fall Creek by boiling water from this source or using bottled water from private vendors. A resident of one of the towns bordering Fall Creek even offered to sell Cornell "adequate and pure" artesian well water at a cheap price if university officials would continue to overlook their use of the creek as a sewer for their sinks, tubs, and water closets.[38]

By 1903, Ithaca was ripe for an epidemic of typhoid fever or some other waterborne disease, and male Cornell students were among the most vulnerable because of their age and their off-campus living conditions. In late January of that year, the first signs of trouble began to appear. The Ithaca papers reported that seventy-three residents of the city were ill with "Ithaca fever." On 23 January, the first student with the illness entered the Cornell Infirmary. Because some degree of intestinal illness was common among students, university officials remained unconcerned until the first week in February, when thirty students were admitted to the infirmary within the span of a few days. That week, Dr. Veranus A. Moore of the Cornell Veterinary College administered a diagnostic blood test to several patients with the "prevailing fever" and found each to be a case of typhoid. The number of cases grew at an alarming rate: a week later, the infirmary had fifty-two typhoid patients, and the number in the city as a whole topped three hundred. On 14 February, when the number of cases in the city neared five hundred, the state department of health sent its expert on infectious disease, Dr. F. C. Curtis, to investigate the situation. After spending a day observing the conditions in Ithaca, Curtis reported to state commissioner of health Daniel Lewis that the disease was undoubtedly typhoid and attributed the source of outbreak to water supplied by the Ithaca Water Works Company. Curtis advised citizens to boil city water before use, reassuring them that the epidemic would soon die down.[39]

Despite Curtis's attempts to control the epidemic and soothe Ithaca's residents, matters grew steadily worse. By the third week in February, the city population and university community were in a state of panic. New cases of typhoid appeared at a rate of twenty or more a day. The Cornell University Infirmary proved inadequate to meet the demands of the epidemic, so the university acquired additional buildings to house the overflow of patients. Cornell hired extra nurses from New York City, Rochester, and other local cities and towns to care for the students in the infirmary and its annexes.[40] Dozens of Cornell students left the university each day because of illness or at the request of their parents. By 18 February, nearly a quarter of the twenty-two hundred students had left for home, and fully one-third of the student population withdrew from the university during February and March.[41]

Soon after the epidemic began, various factions within the city and the university community began looking for someone to bear the blame for the tragedy. The chief target of popular criticism was the privately owned Ithaca Water Works Company. Many Ithacans had long been suspicious of this "corrupt" big business. This mistrust was confirmed at the height of the 1903 epidemic, when Cornell University scientists found evidence of typhoid bacilli in both Six Mile and Buttermilk Creeks.[42]

The 1903 epidemic also resonated with long-standing class and ethnic prejudices within the city, as rumors circulated that a possible source of the typhoid contamination was a group of Italian and Hungarian workers who were constructing a dam for the Ithaca Water Works Company on Six Mile Creek. During the epidemic, the local papers were full of lurid accounts of the allegedly filthy habits of these foreigners, often referring to them as the source of typhoid infection even though none of the health officers appointed to investigate the epidemic found any evidence of disease among the workers. Several professors from Cornell's botany department, however, noted that the immigrant workers washed their clothes in Six Mile Creek and relieved themselves along its banks. Although these accusations arouse in part out of bad feelings toward the water company, the fact that these workers were immigrants certainly had something to do with middle-class Ithacans' willingness to lay blame for city's misfortunes.[43]

Cornell University also became a target of suspicion because of close financial and professional ties with the Ithaca Water Works Company. Several members of the university's department of engineering served as consultants for the water company's various construction projects, and the university owned approximately one hundred thousand dollars' worth of bonds in the company. Numerous rumors appeared in the local press about Cornell's alleged "conspiracy" with the water company. Cornell's most formidable adversary was the *Ithaca Daily News*, the official paper of Ithaca's Democratic Party, which copied the muckraking journalistic style of many other Progressive Era newspapers. The *News* attacked Cornell scientists for failing to foresee the epidemic. Reporters even suggested that knowledge of contamination had been purposely suppressed to protect the university's financial interests in the water company.[44]

Cornell administrators and alumni, trying to divert suspicion away from the university, called attention to Ithaca taxpayers' apathy toward municipal reform before the epidemic. Alumnus Justus L. Barnes, for example, pointed out many of the civic improvements already in effect at Ithaca might never have come about "but for the active support and intervention of the splendid men [the Cornell trustees] who from the beginning have stood by the university and benefited the town."[45]

However, university officials could not entirely free themselves from blame. Although they had little control over the city or campus water supply, the university's response to the outbreak failed to meet the expectations of both parents and students. Despite the mass exodus of students from the city, President Schurman refused to close the university, believing that doing so would cause "no end of harm" by greatly exaggerating the extent of the epidemic. Instead, Schurman kept the university open and declared that "no expense" would be spared to "make the college community as healthful as possible."[46] As a short-term solution to the campus water supply, Schurman made sure that all university buildings were supplied with bottled artesian well water. Andrew Carnegie, one of the university's trustees and a victim of typhoid fever as a child, offered to pay for the cost of installing the filtration plant for the campus water supply. After the plant was completed during the summer of 1903, the head of the toxicology department, Chamot, had the "honor" of reporting on the "absolute purity" of the water it supplied.[47]

In early April, Carnegie extended his generosity to the students who had been ill during the epidemic, offering to pay all their medical expenses and place each one "in precisely the same pecuniary condition as that which he occupied at the outbreak of the epidemic." Carnegie also agreed to pay for the expenses incurred by the parents of students who had lost their lives during the epidemic.[48] Carnegie's actions were possibly an attempt to bolster Cornell's image as an egalitarian institution, since it made it possible for low-income students who contracted typhoid to stay in school. However, Carnegie refused to extend this generosity across racial lines. For example, he refused to reimburse a Puerto Rican student for his medical expenses, claiming that he probably contracted the disease in his mother's home in Manhattan rather than in Ithaca.[49]

Schurman also made some effort to protect male students off campus by appointing a state health official to inspect all boardinghouses inhabited by Cornell students. He also asked boardinghouse keepers to sign a pledge promising to abide by health department recommendations to boil all city water before use. These measures appear to have been poorly enforced, since students claimed to observe numerous health violations even within homes that had agreed to follow Schurman's orders. On 18 February, members of the junior and senior classes demanded the board of trustees take more radical action by furnishing boardinghouses with bottled drinking water at the university's expense, but the trustees refused the request. In a *Cornell Daily Sun* editorial, one student condemned this decision, noting that while trustees could oversee the sanitary conditions of their own homes, Cornell men were forced to rely on boardinghouse keepers "whose interests in our welfare are purely financial."[50]

The following day, President Schurman defended the trustees' decision in an address to the students on the "Present Conditions." Schurman claimed the students' request was financially and logistically impractical. For those who could not trust their boardinghouse keepers to use bottled water, Schurman agreed set up a dining hall for men at Sage gymnasium that could accommodate three hundred students, a small portion of the male student body. Yet Schurman concluded his speech by placing the ultimate responsibility for prevention on the shoulders of Cornell men: "The Trustees have felt that every student should be the guardian of his own health. . . . We have done the utmost in our power to protect the University and the students; the rest is in your hands."[51]

This emphasis on personal choice and responsibility extended to those who chose to leave the university. During the third week of February, Schurman announced to students and their parents that "no reflection will be cast upon any student who leaves," and all students who did so would be allowed to make up their work upon their return with no damage to their academic standing. Schurman added that while a few students had come back to college, "the University advises no students to return: each must decide for himself in view of the facts of the case."[52]

One satirical article from the 3 March 1903 issue of the *Ithaca Daily News* suggested that Cornell was more interested in protecting its image and finances than in preserving student health. A variation on the popular "Mr. Dooley" political satires created by Finley Peter Dunne, the article depicted a character named Hooley telling his friend, Hinnissy, that at Cornell "if the byes dhrink whiskey and git dhrunk the faculty fires 'em, but if they dhrink the wather and die the faculty . . . fergives thim. 'Tis so comfortin' to the parents, Hinnissy, to know the byes is not dhrunkards."[53]

The mixed signals from the Cornell administration upset many parents, who felt that Schurman and the trustees were preserving the university's image at the expense of student safety. The most pressing issue for many parents was the housing policy for female students, which made it clear that only male students were capable of being guardians of their own health. Many parents did not believe their sons had the knowledge or experience to make decisions about their own health. Instead, these parents insisted that the university play a stronger role protecting Cornell men. Mrs. W. U. Bateman, for example, wrote to President Schurman that she was "very particular" about her son's health. She wanted help in finding a boardinghouse where he would be surrounded by other respectable young men in their late teens who had "good morals and clean, pure habits." Mrs. Bateman added, "I should not hesitate as to price, the health and congenial surroundings being paramount to the price."[54] U.S. Navy commander Edward L. Prime of Huntington, New York, who lost his only son to the epidemic, expressed his outrage at Carnegie's offer to pay his son's medical and funeral expenses, calling the compensation "blood money," an "insult" that "looked like a sop to keep my mouth shut." Prime asked Schurman, "How would you have looked at it if the case had been your son? Perhaps judging from the way matters went at Cornell," Prime wrote bitterly, Schurman would have been "very glad to have accepted it thus putting a money value on your children."[55]

Such letters reflected attitudes about the "pricelessness" of children and adolescents that were becoming increasingly common in the early twentieth century, even among parents of working-class children who needed their income to support the family. Indeed, the expansion of higher education and the growth of learned professions made some working-class parents willing to forgo a child's wages so he or she could have a better chance at a middle-class life. This new perspective on children and youth was reflected in the changing practices of life insurance companies and their clients. Rather than insure a child against lost wages or to pay for a decent burial, many parents bought "nest eggs" to pay for a child's higher education so that they had a better chance at upward social mobility.[56]

Parents' letters also illustrate major changes in their perceptions about the duty of colleges and universities toward student health, particularly that of male students. For decades, parents expected that colleges and universities would preserve the health and morality of their daughters. Reactions to the Cornell typhoid epidemic of 1903 indicate that parents believed the university should adopt the same role in loco parentis for Cornell men. Parents' concerns about their sons' health frequently carried overtones of sexual danger: like Mrs. Bateman, parents believed that the university had the responsibility not only to educate their sons but to make sure that they adopted morally pure habits as well.

Pressure from parents finally convinced the trustees to consider constructing dormitories for Cornell men. During the summer of 1903, construction began on Sheldon Court, designed to house one hundred men.

At the same time, the university decided to set up several cafeterias for male students, which served food and drink that received the same sanitary oversight as Sage College. The cafeterias were tremendously popular among male students, who found the food cheaper, better, and "safer" than that served at their boardinghouses.[57]

However, university officials and parents alike came up against a major roadblock in their attempts to protect men's health: male Cornellians themselves. Although Sheldon Court could not begin to meet the housing needs of the two thousand men who attended Cornell, the new dormitory was seldom filled to capacity during its first two decades of operation. Students frequently complained about the expense of room and board at the dormitory. More importantly, male students were reluctant to subject themselves to the same level of surveillance endured by female students at Sage College. Because of the lukewarm reception to Sheldon Court, the university did not begin to build additional housing for the men until nearly ten years after the epidemic.[58] Instead of forcing male students to reside in closely supervised dormitories, the best the university could do was to clean up the city of Ithaca and hope male students would make the right choices to guard their own health.

Female Cornellians did not receive the same options: the residency requirement for women students remained in place until the mid-1960s. At the same time, dormitory space for women fell far short of the number of qualified female students who wished to attend Cornell. Consequently, female enrollment did not exceed 25 percent until after parietal rules were removed in the 1960s.[59] Therefore, a policy that was originally designed to protect the moral and physical health of college women eventually restricted their access to the university, since female admissions were limited by the availability of dormitory space. This pattern became typical at other coeducational institutions as well. Indeed, the controversy over female higher education precipitated by Dr. Edward Clarke's book ensured that women at coeducational institutions lacked the same freedoms as college men. Developments in public health would soon redirect preventive efforts toward the individual student body and personal risk factors rather than the broad programs of environmental sanitary reform that were popular during the Progressive Era.

Medical Screening and Sorting

Rather than providing a safe environment for male students, colleges and universities preferred to screen out those whom they felt were too delicate to withstand the strains of collegiate life. Monitoring individual student bodies was one purpose of the anthropometric measurements conducted by physicians and physical educators interested in examining the impact of exercise on the physique. By the early twentieth century, these physical examinations began to serve a screening function as well, much as they did for job applicants and immigrants arriving at Ellis Island and other points of entry to the United States.[60] Harvard president Charles W. Eliot, for example, claimed that poor health among students resulted largely from a "singular notion" that "feeble, sickly children . . . should be sent to school and college, since they are apparently unfit for hard work." Eliot argued that this practice was foolhardy, since attainment of success in college and the professions required an "extraordinary toughness of body [that] must accompany extraordinary mental powers." Instead of allowing the unfit to waste college resources, Eliot and other college administrators at this time preferred to deny admission to students who could not demonstrate good health prior to admission.[61]

The women's colleges too preferred to exclude rather than rehabilitate sickly student bodies. Annah May Soule of Mount Holyoke argued that physicians should ensure college resources were "as carefully invested as the manager of a factory [sees] that the money he has is wisely invested in a machine." Although one "cannot run a college on the basis of a factory," she admitted, "that does not mean that we are not to be as conscientious in the expenditure as we would be if we were running a factory." Since "our stores and factories are demanding well-proportioned, healthy workers," Soule concluded, "it would seem that our schools could demand no less."[62]

Frequently these efforts to eliminate "unfit" bodies were intertwined with quota systems designed to limit the enrollment of Jewish students, whose bodies were believed to be inferior to those of the white, native-born middle classes. At Dartmouth College, for example, applicants were required to include a photograph so that Jewish students "of a physical type that is unattractive to the average Dartmouth student" could be excluded.[63]

This level of exclusion was not as prevalent at state institutions, which faced pressure from taxpayers to admit all students who were qualified for advanced study. Nevertheless, state institutions did attempt to screen out those whom they believed posed serious threats to the health of other students. They also required that students be vaccinated against major contagious diseases such as diphtheria and smallpox.[64]

At the same time, many colleges and universities became concerned with issues of "wasted manpower." This desire to reduce "human wastage" drew on concepts from the conservation movement of the late nineteenth and early twentieth centuries. The most prominent leader of the conservation movement was President Theodore Roosevelt, who advocated preservation of open spaces to provide all young men with opportunities for a "strenuous life" that would preserve not only their health but their manliness as well. Psychologist G. Stanley Hall also promoted outdoor recreation as a way to recapitulate "primitive" stages of human development, thereby compensating for the "feminizing" influences of modern urban industrial society. Conservation efforts initially sought to protect the landscapes in which bodies could recreate and rejuvenate.[65]

By the early 1910s, the same metaphors of conservation were being directed at bodies themselves. Like their counterparts in industry, insurance, and immigrant medical inspection, physicians on campus were asked to address "competing claims," which demanded exclusion of incurables who would be permanently dependent on state support yet identification of salvageable bodies that could be shaped to suit the manpower needs of the expanding U.S. economy.[66] Institutions of higher education began to employ physicians not only to direct physical education programs and teach hygiene classes but also to control absenteeism by distinguishing between students who were absent from class because they were truly ill and those who were simply "malingerers."[67] In 1893, the Harvard Corporation created the position of "medical visitor" for this purpose, stipulating that the visitor was not to practice for money among the students but could give "gratuitous advice about diet, sleep, exercise, and work, to students who ask it of him." The medical visitor's main responsibilities were to verify that students had genuine illnesses, to ensure that students had proper medical attention from a local physician, and to see that contagious cases were removed from student houses and placed in one of the local hospitals.[68]

At the University of California, the men's physician, George F. Reinhardt, recalled that his position owed "its existence less to a direct effort to improve student health than an effort to improve class attendance." In 1900, faculty asked for an investigation into the causes of escalating student absences, hoping to mete out strict discipline to chronic delinquents. In response to these concerns, university president Benjamin Ide Wheeler appointed a university board of health to oversee the sanitary condition of the campus, hiring Reinhardt to teach hygiene classes and serve as medical adviser to male students. Dr. Mary Bennett Ritter continued to serve as medical adviser to the women students. Both physicians soon found "sickness and not idleness or lack of interest" were the cause of most student absences.[69]

College physicians deliberately used industrial medicine and other forms of contract practice as templates for a new branch of preventive medical practice aimed at the college-age population. The term *contract practice* referred to a system in which a physician would, in exchange for a fixed fee per annum, provide unlimited medical care to a group of patients, such as those belonging to mutual aid societies, fraternal lodges, factories, logging camps, ranches, slave plantations, and other places of employment. As early as the 1860s, Edward Hitchcock Jr. suggested the adoption of this system at Amherst. Like most male colleges, Amherst expected students to seek medical care on their own outside the college. Hitchcock was hired to direct the program in physical education, not to serve as a physician in attendance to the students. However, Hitchcock became a trusted medical adviser for many students. Thus, from the beginning of his appointment, students began to consult him for various illnesses and physical complaints. Even though it was not part of his official duties, Hitchcock felt obligated to attend to their medical needs. As Hitchcock reported to the trustees after his first year of service, he attended each and every case of illness among the students "as often as I thought a Physician should visit his patient whether he has been visited by another Physician or not. In fully three-fourths of the cases I have been the only medical person who has attended them, and I have made it a point to visit sick students daily, that the Government of College might know the condition of its students, and also guard against spurious or vicious sickness."[70] By the end of the 1860s, Hitchcock was using the U.S. Sanitary Commission as a model for health care delivery for male students.[71]

Hitchcock's suggestions were hindered by opposition from the mainstream medical profession. In 1869, the American Medical Association first condemned contract practice as "contrary to medical ethics," since contract physicians frequently undercut the fees charged by physicians in private practice, and resolved that physicians who entered into such contracts "be classified as irregular practitioners." Despite opposition from the American Medical Association and local medical groups, contract practice became increasingly common in the late nineteenth and early twentieth centuries, particularly in urban areas inhabited by immigrant workers and their families who could not afford traditional fee-for-service medical care.[72]

By the early twentieth century, physicians at the nation's colleges and universities were following the example of contract practice. Robert T. Legge, who succeeded Reinhardt as director of the student infirmary at Berkeley, drew on his experience as a contract physician for a Northern

California lumber company to justify creating similar arrangements for college students. Legge observed that the demand for contract service had expanded with the country's commercial activities, "so that now few great manufacturing concerns where large numbers of employees are centered are without a service of this kind." Legge believed such a trend was "fitting entirely the purposes of social evolution," since it not only has "brought about universal propaganda for a legislative health-insurance system" but also has created demand for similar forms of group practice in other venues.[73] Forsythe too suggested that the "more recent general emphasis placed upon group or social health and preventive medicine" in other occupational and social groups "has doubtless added to the desirability of college supervision of student health."[74]

The majority of the mainstream medical profession, however, did not agree that college students needed doctors of their own. Therefore, the creation of student medical services and infirmaries depended heavily on location. Cornell had established a student infirmary before the 1903 epidemic, and during the crisis, President Schurman declared "nothing shall be spared" to obtain medical care for the university's sick.[75] The university added dozens of new beds to the infirmary, increased the number of physicians and nurses on the health service staff, and built laboratories for diagnosing and treating student illnesses. By the time of World War I, Cornell could boast that its health service was one of the nation's best.[76]

Other colleges and universities were slower to create health services for students, but not because these institutions were unconcerned with student health. At rural campuses where medical institutions and practitioners were scarce, college health services faced little opposition and quickly established themselves as centers of medical expertise not only for students but also for faculty, their families, and members of the surrounding community. As Princeton Health Service director Joseph E. Raycroft observed, "Since the health interests of the university are closely bound up with those of the town, a natural and harmonious relationship has grown up between these two parts of the community for the promotion of the general health."[77]

Colleges and universities located in areas with a surplus of medical professionals tended to encounter more tensions with local physicians groups. When the University of Wisconsin established a student health service in 1902, local physicians condemned the university's actions as "a step toward socialized medicine."[78] Likewise, at the University of Kansas, campus physician John Sundwall reported the "relation to the local medical profession" gave the university health service their "most serious difficulties."

To overcome these conflicts, the university did not directly provide health care but rather referred students to local physicians "in whom the service has full confidence."[79]

Off-campus medical care varied considerably in quality and in price. Students with limited resources were often forced to drop out because of untreated health problems. This fact prompted some students to create self-help organizations to finance health services for less fortunate classmates. Modeling themselves after insurance programs offered by fraternal organizations such as the Odd Fellows and Freemasons, some early-twentieth-century student organizations began to create health care funds for students who could not otherwise afford medical care.[80] The first such student-run health benefit societies emerged in California, a state where social insurance programs sponsored by labor unions and mutual aid organizations were especially prevalent. One of the earliest student organizations dedicated specifically to providing a kind of prepaid health insurance was the Students' Guild, established at Stanford University in 1895. Although Stanford officials had hired Dr. Thomas D. Wood to head the Department of Hygiene and Physical Education and Clelia Duel Mosher to oversee the health of women students shortly after the university opened in 1891, their responsibilities in the gymnasium and the hygiene classroom left little time for actual medical treatment of student illnesses. There were no hospital facilities in neighboring towns: students requiring hospitalization had to return to their homes or go to San Francisco or Oakland for treatment. In 1894, students and faculty held a mass meeting to discuss the need for more systematic provision of medical services, and in February 1895, the Students' Guild was founded as a mutual aid society to provide financial aid to members when they were sick. Membership in the guild entitled students to "simple remedies" and "sickroom care" by a trained nurse. Since fewer than half the university's students joined, the guild could not provide coverage for physician fees and hospitalization. In 1903, a devastating outbreak of typhoid fever in Palo Alto taxed the guild's resources even further as it extended services to all students and rented a building in Palo Alto to serve as a makeshift hospital for those who fell ill. The guild subsequently created a hospital for students on the campus and raised membership fees to make up for the expenses of expanded medical care. However, collection of dues proved so troublesome that the university eventually assumed fiduciary control of the guild and made the health fee mandatory in 1906. Opposition from physicians and laypersons in the surrounding community was swift. Physicians in Palo Alto accused Stanford of monopolizing health care for students, while laypersons and physicians alike warned of the dangers of housing a hospital for contagious diseases within the city limits.[81] As a result of this opposition, Stanford did not allow the medical advisers to administer health care to the students and referred students needing hospital care to facilities in San Francisco.[82]

At the University of California, a progressive spirit among students, faculty, and members of the Berkeley community paved the way for the creation of the health service. In 1902, following the discovery of two cases of smallpox in a Berkeley restaurant frequented by university students, President Wheeler approved a recommendation from the University Board of Health advising that all students be vaccinated against the disease.[83] After five cases were found at the university itself in 1904, Wheeler authorized a measure requiring that all students entering the university be satisfactorily vaccinated. Such measures were not universally popular: in fact, California had a strong antivaccination movement that tried unsuccessfully to make allowances for students if they or their parents objected to vaccination.[84]

More importantly, vaccination did nothing to prevent or manage other communicable diseases, such as influenza, gastrointestinal complaints, and upper respiratory infections that were much more common in the student population. To meet this need, benevolent organizations founded the Berkeley Hospital Association to raise funds to build a new public hospital in Berkeley.[85] The Prytanean Society, an honor society for women students, contributed to this effort by collecting money to endow a room for the use of students. Modeled after the Golden Bear Honor Society, which refused to admit women, the Prytanean Society was founded in 1900 by a group of female students eager to be of service to their alma mater. The founding members included two pre-medical students, Romilda Paroni and Ruby Cunningham, who would go on to serve in the college infirmary, and Dr. Ritter, who served as faculty adviser.[86] Ritter recalled that the most pressing need for female students was a place for them to go for rest and treatment when they were sick."[87] Reinhardt agreed that the same was true for male students, since those with communicable diseases were denied admission to private hospitals in Berkeley. Rather than traveling to the state-run hospital in Oakland, students remained in their rooms, "where proper attention is impossible, and where the risks of illness are intensified." Poor health was especially prevalent among students of limited means who had to work to support themselves and who were forced to live in the least expensive accommodations in Berkeley and surrounding towns. These students were more likely to become ill, since they were so poorly nourished they could not resist disease. Even students with better economic circumstances had few options when they fell sick since there was nowhere in the city that would accept them for hospital care. Moreover, Reinhardt noted, most housekeepers did not want the bother of caring for sick students, nor would they accept the disruption to household routine caused by the presence of private nurses. The result was "any student sick and away from home fails to receive such care and attention as public policy demands." Reinhardt pointed to the example of more progressive institutions, such as Princeton, Cornell, and the University of Alabama, which provided infirmaries regardless of cost. Reinhardt observed that even the poorest students at Berkeley were willing to pay a small fee to support an infirmary where they could receive appropriate care when ill. Reinhardt concluded that the creation of such a service "would be an immense relief to the mind of every student of limited resources, a great comfort to all parents, and the means of saving many lives."[88]

Lack of interest among the majority of city residents, combined with fears about housing a hospital for contagious diseases within the city limits, forced the Berkeley Hospital Association to abandon its plans for a city hospital. Instead, the association gave the funds to Prytanean and other student leaders to further their efforts to build an infirmary on campus.[89] Prytanean co-founder Adele Lewis Grant recalled that Wheeler had recently come from Cornell and so was convinced of the value of a student infirmary but that "the Regents were opposed to it, very definitely."[90] In addition, as elsewhere, efforts to create a health service faced considerable opposition from Berkeley's medical community, which, like physicians elsewhere, condemned the plan as an "unethical" form of "socialized medicine." Even some members of the faculty were skeptical about providing health service, believing it was not part of a university's role.[91] Despite the student newspaper's urgent pleas for a hospital, not until the earthquake of 1906 did the regents finally approve plans for a student infirmary. Although Berkeley escaped with only minor damage, the presence of thousands of earthquake survivors from Oakland and San Francisco, including students and their families, on and around the university's campus drove home the need for a health care facility there.[92]

At the University of Minnesota, following a 1904 typhoid epidemic in the southeastern part of the state, students requested that a "sickness fund" be created to pay for medical and hospital care for students who became ill. The regents refused to approve the measure but appointed a university health committee to oversee public health matters on campus. These activities eventually came to include inspecting the safety of the water supply, including the swimming pool, free smallpox and typhoid vaccinations for students, and courses in hygiene.[93]

For black students, segregation and racial discrimination proved formidable barriers to healthy living and decent health care. At Howard University, a shortage of health care facilities that served blacks meant that even middle-class students suffered higher rates of serious diseases than did white youth. Segregation in the District of Columbia also meant that Howard students frequently had difficulty finding suitable housing that met minimal modern standards of health and safety.[94]

Yet as more and more institutions of higher education attempted to follow the example of Cornell, Princeton, and California, they were forced to find ways to defend themselves against opposition from physicians in private practice. During the decades following World War I, physicians in college health sought to prove that they were more than "company doctors," making a self-conscious effort to upgrade their field by establishing special claims to knowledge that other physicians lacked.

CHAPTER 4

Neither a Commonwealth nor a Corporation

In June 1927, an editorial in the *American Medical Association Bulletin* roundly condemned a "plan of organization of medical service for students in educational institutions" under which each student paid a nominal annual fee in exchange for unlimited dispensary and infirmary care. The editorial described these kinds of plans as "a most obnoxious form of contract practice" that offered at best "cut-rate" medical service. What made college health services particularly troublesome was the clientele: relatively well-to-do students to whom a college was "under no more obligation to supply medical care" than it was "to supply clothing, food or any other necessities."[1]

As the previous chapter demonstrated, the opposition by the American Medical Association (AMA) to this "obnoxious" form of contract practice originated with the first college health services at the turn of the century. The battle against "socialized medicine"—a term applied to all forms of group practice, not just those sponsored by state or federal funds—gained ground in the conservative political environment of the 1920s. The Red Scare following the Bolshevik Revolution as well as President Warren G. Harding's call for a "return to normalcy" after the country's involvement in World War I undercut public support for Progressive Era social reforms. By the mid-1920s, the AMA had launched a campaign against the 1921 Sheppard-Towner Maternity and Infancy Act, which had allocated federal dollars to state health centers providing free health care to indigent women and children.[2]

To combat the AMA's opposition, physicians in college health presented themselves as more than merely "company doctors." As Dr. H. E. Robertson of the University of Minnesota argued at a conference on school health in 1914, a health service at an institution of higher education was "neither a commonwealth nor a corporation, although sharing in the characteristics of both." Robertson argued that public health measures adopted by towns, cities, states, and the federal government were insufficient for the needs of university, as were methods adopted by business and industry. Even the principles of school hygiene, Robertson claimed, were ill suited to higher education, "for the university cannot be likened to a public school; it is *sui generis*, and many fallacies in our entire educational system might become more readily apparent if these distinctions were given their proper recognition."[3] As the number of college health programs grew, college physicians attempted to improve their professional image by redefining the scope and goals of their field and more firmly grounding college health in the principles of scientific medicine. Demonstrating the unique features of college health services required the creation of a new professional organization with a mission distinct from other branches of public health. At the center of these efforts to legitimize college health programs was a particular definition of the student as patient and the college environment as a locus of medical practice.

Engendering a Scientific Spirit

On 4–5 March 1920, University of Minnesota Health Service Director John Sundwall brought together twenty individuals involved in student health work to plan creating a new professional organization called the American Student Health Association. (In 1948, the name of this organization was changed to the American College Health Association [ACHA]. We will refer to the organization as ACHA throughout.) In his keynote address at the association's first annual meeting that December, held in conjunction with the National Collegiate Athletic Association and various physical education societies, Sundwall declared that the creation of the new organization had been prompted in part by the "appalling results of the nation's attempts to raise an army for the world war," as between 25 and 30 percent of college-age young men were rejected for service. Sundwall acknowledged the work of pioneering physical educators such as Edward Hitchcock Jr., "for those interested in physical education have always been interested in students' health." However, Sundwall also argued, "great advancement in the various sciences making up modern medicine" required the formation of a new organization incorporating not only physical exercise but also oversight of diet, rest, personal hygiene, and various other factors that contributed "far more to the 'break down' than does neglect of exercise."[4] Although physical educators, coaches, and athletic directors were allowed to participate in the ACHA, physicians in the organization adamantly distinguished between their work as *medical* professionals and that of physical educators and coaches. Of the fifty-three individuals who signed the ACHA constitution during its first year, only thirteen listed physical education as their professional appointment.[5]

The creation of the ACHA represented a generational shift in the focus of college health programs as well as the training of those who directed them. According to the organization's secretary-treasurer, Warren Forsythe, health services at American colleges and universities were in the process of evolving from an early "gymnastic period," which emphasized physical education and anthropometry, to a "period of health promotion," which fused curative medicine, public health, physical education, and hygiene teaching under a single university health department headed by medical doctors.[6] This move resulted partly from changes in the training of those involved in physical education and college athletics. Although late-nineteenth-century physical educators usually had medical degrees, by the early twentieth century physical educators more commonly received their training in departments of physical education at state universities and normal schools. Coaches and athletics trainers were even less likely to have medical degrees. In some cases, they lacked physical education training as well. The result was a growing professional divide between an earlier generation of college health professionals whose emphasis was physical education and the younger generation represented by the ACHA's founding members, who were trained in public health and preventive medicine. Influenced by the "new public health" that grew out of the bacteriological discoveries of the early twentieth century, this new era of college health increasingly focused on individual health care and hygiene education rather than on the physical education programs that had dominated previous efforts to protect the health of student bodies.[7]

This emphasis on the "new public health" meant that directors of college health programs should be medical doctors trained in the most up-to-date methods of preventive medicine and personal hygiene. The benefits of a well-trained medical staff on campus were driven home by the influenza epidemic of 1918–19, which took its greatest toll on adolescent and young adult males.[8] Even institutions with long-established infirmaries used the epidemic to justify an expansion of health care services. At Princeton, the Women's Committee of the Princeton Endowment Fund observed that while the university had not experienced a single death in the 192 influenza cases seen at the infirmary, the epidemic had strained the facility to capacity. Committee members also noted that the growth in the number of students further rendered the current infirmary inadequate.[9]

Sundwall's background exemplified this transition from physical education to the new public health. He had both a doctorate (1906) in anatomy and pathology from the University of Chicago, a leading graduate program in that field at the time, and a medical degree (1912) from Johns Hopkins University. After spending a few years as a hygiene expert and assistant surgeon with the U.S. Public Health Service, he accepted a joint appointment as professor of anatomy and director of the health service at the University of Kansas. Sundwall's exemplary work in medicine and public health soon led to the offer of a position as professor of anatomy and dean of medical sciences at the University of Illinois. However, U.S. entry into World War I led him to decline the offer and instead enter the Reserve Officer Training Corps at Fort Sheridan in June 1918. Sundwall hoped to serve with the American Expeditionary Forces overseas, but his work at Kansas was so well known that president Marion LeRoy Burton of the University of Minnesota invited Sundwall to establish and direct the health services of the Student Army Training Corps on that campus.[10] Burton's earlier work as president of Smith College had convinced him of the necessity of providing health care and preventive medicine for female students. He therefore felt that providing a similar service to male and female students alike was "indispensable" to running a large institution like the University of Minnesota.[11] In March 1918, Burton convinced the regents to commit five thousand dollars of the university budget to creating an infirmary for all students, with students paying three dollars per semester as a health fee.[12] On 24 July, the regents approved Sundwall's appointment as head of the new health service. Years later, Burton wrote, "There seemed something almost providential about getting the Health Service started just in time to serve during that pandemic."[13] According to Sundwall, during the first year of operation, the health service saw two thousand cases of influenza—eight hundred of them civilian students—with twenty deaths.[14]

In 1921, when Burton became president of the University of Michigan, he invited Sundwall to come with him to Ann Arbor. Although Sundwall believed he was accomplishing more at Minnesota than he had been able to do at Kansas, the offer to go to Michigan was appealing because Burton insisted on a "sharp line of demarcation" between Sundwall's position and intercollegiate athletics. Sundwall and athletic director Fielding Yost would have the same administrative status, with neither subordinate to the other. Furthermore, Sundwall would hold the rank of full professor, be a member of the University Senate, and would direct a new Department of Student Welfare that included supervision not only of the health service but also of intramural sports, physical education, and the educational activities of hygiene and public health for the students.[15]

The increasing split between medical professionals and physical educators was exacerbated by the escalating controversy over the dangers of college athletics. Sundwall argued that physical education had become contaminated by the elitism and obsession with winning that permeated sports competitions. Although originally conceived as a health measure, physical education had become "almost entirely engrossed in the tecnic of performance," especially in institutions where intercollegiate athletics had become "a dominating interest in college and university life." The chief role of these programs, observed Sundwall, was not healthful exercise for all but "the gratification of certain innate, powerful, fundamental instincts for physical emulation, competition, rivalry, and mastery." Although some students fulfilled these impulses through competition, most were content to sit comfortably on the sidelines and cheer their team to victory.[16]

Even those whose training was primarily in physical education expressed dissatisfaction with the growing dominance of intercollegiate athletics at the expense of the health of the average student. In correspondence with Sundwall, A. D. Browne, medical adviser of men at Stanford, wrote that repeated football defeats by California's Wonder Team had led the alumni members of the board of control to hire a new head coach as an expert in "physical education," with the duty of studying Stanford's "problems" with beating its rival. The staff had become demoralized, and "no man of any decency" could afford to stay. Browne added that Sundwall was fortunate that his position was not subordinate to the athletics program. At Stanford, where physical education and athletics were inseparably linked, he and his colleagues often found themselves "knocked to pieces" if they failed to satisfy student and alumni expectations for victory.[17]

To more fully distinguish between their mission and those of organizations dedicated to athletics and physical education, ACHA members discussed creating standards for their field. The first challenge was to come up with a common term for comprehensive programs that included all aspects of student health, not just physical education. The thirty-six colleges and universities represented at the ACHA's first meeting, had seventeen different titles for the health work done at these institutions.[18] Sundwall argued that "hygiene and physical education" caused too much "duplication and friction" among various existing departments. Instead, he suggested that the term "student physical welfare," which had been adopted at Michigan, be used to describe all programs that combined physical education, hygiene instruction, health service, and athletics under the direction of a medical doctor. Such vocabulary, Sundwall argued, would not only make these programs distinctive but "give us a concrete example or laboratory in which the problems of public health may be worked out."[19]

Sundwall's use of the word *laboratory* represented attempts to make the field of college health more scientific and hence more in line with other branches of medicine in the early twentieth century. Eugene C. Howe, associate professor of hygiene at Wellesley College, stated that the medical officers of a college or university should do more than deliver care to sick and injured students; they should also "be leaders in adopting the practice of modern medicine" and thereby place "health protection above health salvage." This practice included collecting scientific data showing trends in morbidity. Without this kind of data, Howe argued, the field of college health would remain stuck in an older, prescientific age before vital statistics existed.[20] Harold S. Diehl, director of student health at the University of Minnesota, argued that pursuit of medical research by health center staff would "engender in them a scientific spirit" and make their work less monotonous. Such a staff would be more "progressive" and better able to render high-quality service than those who did nothing but routine duties of running a department.[21] To more firmly establish the distinctiveness of college health, Sundwall suggested that the ACHA cease meeting in conjunction with the physical education directors and the National Collegiate Athletic Association. Meeting with these organizations was fine during the ACHA's infancy, when these were the only organizations that "claimed to have College Health as an objective." Since then, however, the ACHA had "grown up into a sturdy youth able to take care of itself," and the organization should search for affiliates that could help with the problems of the nation's youth. Sundwall urged the ACHA to hold its annual meeting in affiliation with the American Public Health Association, which he believed would "enhance in every way the general scientific spirit of the annual meeting" of the ACHA.[22]

At the same time, members of ACHA argued that college health was also distinctive from other branches of public health and curative medicine. As R. W. Bradshaw of Oberlin College noted, student health "offers opportunities for research found probably nowhere else in the realm of the medical sciences." For that reason, college health should be considered a branch of medicine that offered a unique viewpoint.[23] In short, college health must become a specialty that encompassed features from clinical medicine, public health, and physical education.

A Fairer Chance for Women and African Americans

The ACHA was so intent on emphasizing the medical aspects of its work that the association provided a far more welcoming atmosphere for female physicians than did most other medical organizations at this time. (In fact, many of the more prestigious medical societies banned women entirely.) Like other organizations for public health and preventive medicine at this time, the ACHA was receptive to having women physicians as colleagues.[24] Even nurses were more desirable members of the organization than were physical educators, coaches, and athletic directors, since nurses emphasized health care delivery. Sundwall in particular was extremely supportive of women in the organization. In fact, many of the female students in his hygiene courses went on to become physicians, and he remained a mentor to them throughout their careers.[25]

This level of male support became critical during the Great Depression, as many colleges and universities merged male and female health services in an attempt to cut costs.[26] To justify their role in college health, women physicians continued to argue that female students had special needs and bodily differences that could be addressed only by female physicians. They also upheld female modesty to justify their work, claiming that male physicians should not examine female students. During the late 1920s and early 1930s, women physicians within the ACHA discussed the possibility of holding special sessions on the hygiene of menstruation and menstrual abnormalities as well as on the unique health administration issues of women's colleges.[27] At the same time, women physicians in college health, like professional women more generally, were moving away from separate female institutions.[28] Women insisted that special sessions on female health should not be a precursor to a rival organization for women physicians or even a separate segment within ACHA.[29] Dr. Marjorie Jeffries Wagoner, associate physician at Bryn Mawr, expressed this concern in a letter to ACHA president Warren Forsythe in 1930. Although she agreed that the "problems of particular interest to women's and coeducational colleges should have a place on the regular program," she also saw "no good reason for the women's meeting separately, except informally and for social reasons."[30] Therefore, Wagoner and other women in college health insisted that despite the special concerns of women students, female professionals should have equal status within the ACHA and on the campuses on which they served.

The stature of white women in the ACHA is exemplified by the career of Ruth Evelyn Boynton, who served as executive secretary and in 1940 was elected the organization's first female president. Boynton's background and training ensured that she would be one of the leaders in the emerging field of college health. Her career also illustrates major changes in the outlook of female physicians during the first half of the twentieth century. Boynton was born in La Crosse, Wisconsin, in 1896, the daughter of Ervin and Nellie Alice (Parker) Boynton. When asked what she thought persuaded her to go into medicine, Boynton stated that she was inspired by a husband and wife who served as her family physicians. As was common during that time, the wife in the practice, Dr. Mary P. Houck, mainly treated women and children. She cared for two of Boynton's brothers during their final illnesses and for Boynton's mother, who died while Boynton was in graduate school. Although Houck did not directly encourage Boynton to become a doctor, Boynton was so impressed by the older woman's example that she decided in high school that medicine would be her life's work.[31]

Boynton also benefited from expanding opportunities for female education in the early twentieth century as well as new notions of what it meant to be an educated woman. In 1914, Boynton started her undergraduate work at the University of Wisconsin, which, like many coeducational universities at this time, was trying to adjust to the explosion in female enrollments that occurred during the Progressive Era. Between 1890 and 1920, the number of female undergraduates in the United States grew from 56,000 to 282,900. The greatest growth occurred at coeducational institutions, especially public land-grant universities, where tuition was very inexpensive or nonexistent. By 1920, 81.3 percent of women attended coeducational institutions, most of them public land-grant institutions. At Wisconsin, President Charles Van Hise was committed to coeducation, but like his counterparts at other land-grant institutions, was concerned by the apparent "feminization" of liberal arts as male students abandoned the humanities for other fields. Van Hise believed that part of the problem was that male students disliked having intelligent women as competitors. When he suggested creating single-sex classrooms, he came under vicious attack from both alumnae and their male supporters. Eager to make up for this slip, Van Hise sought to find a new kind of dean of women who would stand in sharp contrast to the "wise and pious matrons" who oversaw the dormitory system for women students. Determined to hire someone who was both a scholar and a seasoned administrator, Van Hise chose Lois Matthews, an associate professor of history at Wellesley and a protégée of University of Wisconsin history professor Frederick Jackson Turner. According to Turner, Matthews was an "exceptional woman in the solidity and masculine quality of her judgment and ability to envisage a question; while she has the essentially womanly qualities that one demands of a woman." Matthews was appointed dean of women and associate professor of history in 1911 and soon demonstrated her determination to make women equal members of the university's intellectual community. Matthews was especially concerned that too many women students judged themselves according to a male standard of "social availability"—that is, physical attractiveness—rather than for their professional or intellectual accomplishments. Matthews also believed in encouraging women students to pursue careers besides the profession of teaching, which was becoming so dominated by women that wages were barely above subsistence levels. To this end, Matthews held vocational conferences where she brought in female professionals from various fields, including journalism, medicine, and library work, as well as Jane Addams and other famous women reformers from Hull House in Chicago. When the United States entered World War I in April 1917, opportunities for women at Wisconsin expanded even further as female undergraduates took over positions in campus organizations that had been vacated by men. Matthews formed the Women's War Work Council to help channel women into new professional opportunities, including medicine and other service professions, which Matthews defined as "Christianity applied to everyday living."[32]

Although Boynton did not comment on her undergraduate experiences, it is likely that studying in an educational environment that encouraged women's intellectual development and commitment to social welfare greatly influenced her choice of career. After completing her bachelor's degree at the University of Wisconsin in 1918, Boynton began her medical studies that fall at the University of Minnesota, another midwestern institution that had recently undergone a fitful adjustment to the growing presence of women on campus. As at Wisconsin, Minnesota's female students profited from the presence of a strong women's dean dedicated to "opening minds and opening doors" for college-educated women.[33] The Minnesota medical school was more welcoming toward female students than other institutions and began admitting a few women shortly after it opened in 1883. In fact, half of the 1887 graduating class was female. Nevertheless,

Minnesota, like other coeducational medical colleges, did not always take women students seriously. Many members of the all-male faculty insinuated that admitting women was a "wasted effort" since most would eventually marry and give up their careers. To create a supportive community for themselves, the female students in 1901 started a chapter of Alpha Epsilon Iota, a national medical fraternity founded at the University of Michigan ten years earlier. The organization sought "to promote good fellowship, to maintain a high order of scholarship and professional achievement," and "to foster a spirit of moral and social helpfulness." Boynton joined Alpha Epsilon Iota while a medical student and strongly supported the organization while a member of the health service staff, helping the organization incorporate in 1944.[34]

Boynton was among the hundreds of students at Minnesota who fell ill with influenza in the fall of 1918. She did not record her memories of the epidemic, but it is likely that her experiences shaped her decision to enter the field of public health. After receiving her M.D. in 1921, new health service director Harold S. Diehl hired Boynton to oversee the health of women students at the university. (Diehl and Charles E. Shepard took care of the male students.) Boynton's first years at the health service were hectic, as the campus experienced successive waves of epidemic influenza, scarlet fever, and smallpox. Severe respiratory infections were also a common problem, as was tuberculosis. To enhance her knowledge and skills in preventive medicine, Boynton pursued advanced graduate training leading to a master's degree in public health, awarded in 1927.[35]

Given her extensive experience and qualifications, Boynton seemed like a natural choice to replace Diehl when he left the health service in 1936 to become dean of the University of Minnesota College of Medical Sciences. Yet Diehl expressed some reservations about promoting Boynton to the directorship. In a letter to President L. D. Coffin, Diehl wrote, "In view of the predominance of male students in the University and male physicians on our staff, I am not certain whether or a woman can satisfactorily administer the department; but if any woman can do it Dr. Boynton will succeed."[36]

Such backhanded compliments were common in an era when women were still struggling to make it in a man's world. Boynton earned the respect of her male colleagues by adopting a male model of professionalism based on scientific medicine and research. At the same time, she distanced herself from women physical educators, whom she considered unqualified to deal with students' medical concerns. Her biographer observes that Boynton had more professional conflicts with the director of physical education for women than with male physicians in the health service. He also praised her for embodying the characteristics "of the good physician with empathy rather than sympathy, objectiveness, and understanding of human nature's nobility and its foibles."[37] In other words, Boynton had discarded traditional notions of feminine "sympathy" toward the sick and adopted modern notions of scientific objectivity.[38] A review of Boynton's extensive publications shows that she carefully balanced her work as a clinician with work as a scientific researcher. Boynton conducted a number of respected studies not only on women's health issues but also on epidemic diseases such as tuberculosis that affected all students. In total, she authored or coauthored more than eighty papers. As a result of these accomplishments, Boynton was elected the ACHA's first female president in 1940. In 1967, the association created the Ruth Boynton Award to honor those who provide distinguished service to the organization.[39]

Equality of opportunity in ACHA stopped short when it came to race, however. Like most medical societies at this time, the ACHA did not admit black practitioners to avoid offending members from whites-only institutions. Instead, black physicians formed a separate organization called the National Student Health Association, the title of which was modeled after the National Medical Association, the black counterpart to the whites-only AMA. Not until Boynton became president were blacks allowed to join ACHA. Despite blacks' exclusion from the ACHA in its early years, Sundwall helped foster the careers of the few African American physicians in college health. His most illustrious protégé was Paul Bertau Cornely, who went on to become a major figure in U.S. public health and civil rights. Cornely was born in Guadeloupe in 1906. After spending his early years in the French West Indies and Puerto Rico, he and his family moved to Detroit in 1920. In 1928, Cornely received a bachelor's degree from the University of Michigan and began medical studies at Michigan's School of Medicine. Like many African Americans at this time, Cornely and his family barely made enough to survive, a condition that worsened during the depression. Cornely recalled that "during my last year in medical school in 1930, I did not know whether or not I would be coming back the following year because there were not jobs available. I did not make the money to help my parents with tuition, books, and other fees like I had been doing in previous years." Fortunately, Michigan had money from the Julius Rosenwald Fund that enabled Cornely and other African American students to complete their medical education. After he received his M.D. in 1931, Cornely's postgraduate training options were limited to black hospitals such as Lincoln Hospital in Durham, North Carolina, where he completed his internship. Unable to find a surgical residency program that would accept a black physician, Cornely returned to Michigan to pursue a degree in public health, again using Rosenwald funds. In 1934, Cornely became the first African American to receive a doctorate in public health.[40]

While at Michigan, Cornely received extensive support from both Forsythe and Sundwall, both of whom were firmly committed to increasing the presence of blacks and women in the college health profession. Cornely worked with Forsythe in the University Health Service while a student in the School of Public Health, an experience that paved his way for Cornely's appointment as director of Howard University's health service in 1937.[41]

Cornely's colleague at Howard, Dorothy Ferebee, illustrates the double burden that sexism and racism imposed on black women in medicine. Like other historically black colleges and universities, Howard provided more opportunities for women professionals than did other institutions. Even at these institutions, however, black women faced sex discrimination and even harassment by male faculty and students.[42] Those black women who succeeded in college health, like their white counterparts, did so by emphasizing the relevance of their work to the health of both male and female students. Like Boynton, Ferebee's success hinged on the support of male mentors who transcended the sexist attitudes of the day. Cornely was foremost among Ferebee's male supporters. As his duties in the College of Medicine and the School of Public Health expanded, Cornely gradually turned over more and more of the daily responsibilities of the health service to Ferebee. Finally, Cornely told Ferebee, "Now you know what Howard University Health Service can do, we want you to take over." In 1949, Cornely left the health service completely to serve as professor in the Howard College of Medicine and head of the Department of Preventive Medicine and Public Health, and Ferebee assumed the directorship of the health service.[43]

Ferebee recalled that her appointment as director prompted a "great deal of jealousy" among male physicians and faculty at Howard, who no doubt resented a woman being promoted to such a position. Fortunately, President Mordecai Wyatt Johnson was a "very staunch ally" who "was absolutely superb" in making sure that both men and women received the recognition they deserved. Ferebee attributed her successful career to Johnson's approval, believing that the few members of the "subterranean faction" that opposed her had little weight given the president's support.[44]

Johnson's endorsement of Ferebee may have been a compensation for the fallout precipitated by his treatment of Dean Lucy Diggs Slowe, who in the 1930s increasingly raised the ire of the president by continually calling for equal opportunity and self-determination for women on campus and by complaining of sexual harassment of female students by male faculty members. Slowe's relationship with longtime companion Mary Burrill, an English teacher at nearby Dunbar High School, probably also contributed to her poor relations with the president, since he like other men at this time became increasingly suspicious of female friendships.[45] The conflict between Slowe and Johnson culminated in 1937, when Slowe became ill (terminally, it turned out) and Johnson ordered her to return to work or lose her job.[46]

Johnson's treatment of Slowe caused an uproar among students and alumni, who were already criticizing Johnson for being a tyrant. Shortly after Slowe's death, the Executive Committee of the Alumni Association issued a pamphlet, *The Case against President Johnson*, in which the committee's members condemned the president's "hate, ill will, and malice" toward the late dean.[47] In the early 1940s, these protests led Johnson to appoint a committee on the status of women at Howard, chaired by history professor Merze Tate. Not surprisingly, the committee found that women were clustered in the lowest ends of the professional ranks and were paid considerably less than men. Johnson's willingness to take some measures to rectify the situation contributed to Ferebee's appointment as director of the health service.[48]

The "chilly climate" for women at Howard made Ferebee willing to cross professional boundaries to improve campus life for women. Unlike Boynton, Ferebee worked well with the chair of the Department of Physical Education for Women, Maryrose Reeves Allen, a fact that could also be attributed to Ferebee's experience as a college athlete. Ferebee believed that Allen's support was instrumental to Ferebee's success as director of the health service and recalled that she and Allen "worked diligently" to make the health service the best it could be given the small amount of money it was allotted.[49] In 1971, the ACHA acknowledged Ferebee's accomplishments by giving her the Edward Hitchcock Award in honor of her outstanding work in advancing the health of college students.

College health thus continued to provide professional opportunities for women physicians in the twentieth century. As in the nineteenth century, the position of college physician gave women physicians one of their few opportunities to serve on the faculty and to be medical researchers. Yet to become heads of department, these women had to show that they could also handle the needs of male students, which accounts for their interest in issues such as infectious and chronic diseases that affected both men and women. Female physicians on college campuses also benefited from other opportunities that opened up for male physicians, many of whom abandoned college health in favor of more prestigious careers in medicine and public health. Boynton reached the rank of full professor at Minnesota and even served as acting director of the School of Public Health while her male colleagues served in the military during the World War II. Yet it is also clear that Boynton encountered the same glass ceiling as did other women physicians and that she had difficulty in achieving her promotion to full faculty rank.[50]

Ferebee's oral history illustrates the added challenges faced by women of color. She realized that she was an exception and was quite outspoken about the discrimination most women faced in academia. Ferebee told an interviewer in 1979 that the Equal Rights Amendment "is as much needed today as it was years ago, because women do not have the recognition or receive the appointments and salaries to which they are entitled."[51] While Ferebee clearly took pride in her accomplishments at Howard, her oral history also conveys the sense that she was disappointed that she did not receive the same level of recognition and status as did Cornely, who after leaving Howard achieved international renown in the field of public health.[52]

Women and blacks proved powerful allies in the struggle for professional legitimacy in college health, as the field fought an ongoing turf war against the mainstream medical profession. Boynton in particular adamantly argued that the ACHA's main purpose was encouraging member institutions to increase the availability of *health* services to its students.[53] The attempts to ally the ACHA with larger trends in scientific medicine helped convince several influential physicians within the AMA to challenge their colleagues' position on college health services.

Campus Health Services and the Committee on the Costs of Medical Care

A key ally in the effort to justify the existence of college health services was Stanford University President Ray Lyman Wilbur, former AMA president and secretary of the interior under President Herbert Hoover. During his time at the AMA's helm, Wilbur had spoken out against the organization's condemnation of "state medicine." In the 1920s, he approved publication of articles on the benefits of college health programs in *Hygeia*, the AMA's journal for a popular audience. At the 1926 AMA convention, a group of like-minded delegates held an informal conference to consider the economic factors affecting the organization of medicine. At the end of the conference, the group appointed the Committee of Five "to formulate a series of studies concerning the economic aspects of medical service, and to develop plans for the creation of a commission which would be responsible for the conduct of these researches by various interested agencies." Among the forms of health care the Committee of Five recommended studying was "the cost per capita of industrial medical service and university health service," which they hoped "would shed much light on the practical possibility of organized medical service, especially if some evaluation of quality and of results could accompany the studies of scope and cost." The committee's secretary, Harry H. Moore of the U.S. Public Health Service, contacted Sundwall at Michigan for input.[54]

The following year, Wilbur presided over a larger discussion of medical economics at the AMA annual convention that resulted in the establishment of a long-range planning group called the Committee on the Cost of Medical Care (CCMC) and dedicated to studying the economic aspects of medical care and prevention of illness. Although the core group consisted of renegade AMA members, the CCMC also included professionals from various public health organizations, hospital administrators, economists, sociologists, and other interested persons within and outside the health care professions. Grants from several private foundations, including the Rockefeller Foundation, the Julius Rosenwald Fund, and the Carnegie Corporation, gave the group nearly a million dollars to finance a five-year study of the "economic aspects of various existing types of medical services," with the "hope that the results of our studies may later point the way to a more efficient organization of medical services in the United States."[55]

Shortly after formation of the CCMC, Sundwall accepted an invitation from the organization's executive committee to direct the study of university health services. The committee was especially eager to study college health centers because they provided a more palatable example of prepayment plans than did those for industrial workers and could serve as a model for prepayment plans for middle-class individuals.[56] In a 1930 letter to Sundwall, committee member Isidore S. Falk wrote that the university study was one of the most desirable for the purposes of the committee's work. Even though funds for the studies were running out, Falk strongly recommended that the university study continue even if it meant ending the other projects.[57] Sundwall sent surveys to six university health services—Cornell, Yale, Michigan, Minnesota, California, and Oregon State—considered the leading examples of group practice for the college age group. The final report concluded that these institutions, along with those of similar scale, were "furnishing medical care of high quality." Furthermore, these services were more efficient than most private practices, since college health personnel were "in a position to concentrate their efforts upon preventive medicine and the early discovery of disease and defects rather than upon remedial measures required to relieve advanced pathological conditions." Most importantly, these health centers had "far-reaching significance" beyond the college campus. Students received "tangible proof of the value of preventive care" that they could carry into their future homes and communities. The student health service's medical personnel were "given an opportunity for research into, and development of, more and more extensive applications of preventive measures into ever widening fields of incipient pathology." Finally, when considered in conjunction with other studies conducted by the CCMC, the survey of university student health centers "may serve to indicate the possibilities inherent in a wider application of the principle of organization for provision of medical care and organization for payment."[58]

The CCMC's executive committee went even further, suggesting that the "organization of university health services and the group-payment by students" should be extended to faculty, staff, and their family members. These services would be "particularly adaptable to institutions conducting medical schools and which are equipped to provide medical care and hospital service for all diseases and conditions," the committee claimed. Such an arrangement, they concluded, "might also tend to improve service and to lower costs to patients in small 'college towns' where the student body and the families of university employees comprise an important section of the population."[59]

Physicians in private practice were outraged by such a proposition, which they considered an illegitimate form of "socialized medicine" for the middle class. Olin West, AMA secretary and general manager, was "disappointed" with Sundwall's work with the CCMC, which West considered an insult to their friendship. "My position is that the benefits of scientific medicine can never be made available for the people except through the instrumentality of a qualified medical profession free from lay or political dictation," West wrote bitterly. "Any scheme that proposes to provide medical services on a machine basis or through any plan of organization that will be operated by governmental agencies will destroy professionalism as surely as it is put into operation."[60] To counter such opposition, college physicians needed to prove that they offered a special form of health care that physicians in private fee-for-service practices were unable or unwilling to provide.

The Health Service as Home

During the early twentieth century, college physicians drew on G. Stanley Hall's latest work on the psychological features of late adolescence to reinforce their position that health services constituted an essential component of institutions of higher education. According to Hall, "One of the last sentiments to be developed in human nature is the sense of responsibility, which is one of the highest and most complex psychic qualities, and in the development of which our carefully nurtured and protected youth of student age, although perhaps more matured in this respect than in any other land, have had little training." Hall argued that male college students needed the same guidance in health matters and medical care as did younger adolescent males.[61]

In an article criticizing the AMA's accusation that college health centers were an "obnoxious form of medical practice," Dr. Seneca Egbert of the University of Pennsylvania made a similar argument, claiming that the university had a responsibility in loco parentis in the area of student health care. Because students leaving home for the first time had little experience in finding doctors, students who became ill tended to avoid seeking medical advice because they feared the verdict or the expense. "For these reasons, if for no others," Egbert claimed, "it would be the positive and moral duty of the educational authorities, to whom the parents have entrusted the physical as well as mental care of their immature sons and daughters, to provide as promptly and conveniently as possible competent medical care and advice for sick students."[62]

College physicians also pointed to the legal responsibility institutions of higher education assumed for students who were far from the protections of home and family. Paul C. Phillips of Amherst College, for example, declared it "doubtful" that when President William Augustus Stearns approved the hygiene department at the college in the 1850s, "any thought of a legal responsibility on the part of the college entered his mind." Since the early twentieth century, however, "there has been an increasing sense of responsibility on the part of American colleges and universities for the health of their students," a characteristic the United States shared with other "civilized nations of the world." Phillips concluded by emphasizing "the moral if not legal responsibility which each college has for providing and maintaining good hygienic conditions for its students." While some observers might argue that "students over 18 years of age should be given the responsibility of care of their own bodies," Phillips contended that "it is a question, however, whether a department of hygiene would be justified in taking this attitude. These students are away from home are given unusual freedom, are under changed conditions and at an age when hygienic living is of great importance to their future."[63]

Sundwall declared the main distinguishing feature of a student health service to be its emphasis on the "preventive aspect, while the hospital is concerned with the curative aspect of medicine." Students were also "young and inexperienced" in negotiating medical institutions and feared dispensary "and particularly hospital treatment." Although by the 1920s hospitals were becoming modern centers of curative medicine, they were still hampered by their older images as institutions of last resort for the destitute.[64] Therefore, like most middle-class Americans, students remained "under the conception that a hospital is a place in which to die, instead of a place in which to get well." Above all, students should not be "intermingled with the average type of hospital patient"—at this time, still impoverished individuals with no family or friends to care for them. Instead, a student health service needed a "hospital of its own" where "the preventive and educational phases of disease may be emphasized" and where a "homelike environment" could be ensured.[65]

This metaphor of the college health center as home was used repeatedly in the series of popular articles for *Hygeia* approved by Wilbur, the AMA's president. "Every college needs a health program," claimed one article, as modern educators were "almost unanimous" in asserting that a college or university was incomplete "unless definite provision is made for the care of the sick and injured students by physicians and trained nurses. Parents should encourage their children to make every use of this service and should themselves find out more about it." D. F. Smiley of Cornell reassured parents that "colleges are taking a real interest in meeting the health needs of the student body" so the graduate will be "in better physical condition with better health up-keep habits than when he entered." Other articles stressed that all "reputable" and "leading" colleges and universities made sure the health care available to students was a good as that available at home. One even touted the notion of "going to college for your health" as becoming the rallying cry of many "modern" institutions of higher learning. Physicians were especially interested in helping preserve and improve the health of students who supported themselves while attending college because they were more prone to illness due to the added strain and fatigue of work and were more likely to avoid seeing a doctor if they had to pay for it themselves. These articles concluded that a health service should be a selling point for an institution, since "parents considering colleges for their children will do well to look to the health departments," just as they would departments of English, history, or other academic disciplines.[66]

Physicians at historically black colleges and universities also emphasized the unique features of college health services as a way of legitimizing their work. Like their counterparts at white institutions, many faculty and administrators at Howard assumed that students could receive all the health care they needed at nearby Freedmen's Hospital, which was affiliated with the university's medical school. The creation of a comprehensive health service formed part of a larger effort to improve the physical environment for students at Howard. This movement intensified after Mordecai Wyatt Johnson became Howard's first black president in 1926. The previous year, a study of the Howard campus indicated that many of the institution's facilities were outdated and even hazardous. Students had already complained about the condition of the athletic facilities and dormitories. Shortly after assuming the presidency, Johnson began a major fund-raising effort, which included appealing to Congress for financial support. In 1928, Congress agreed to give the same appropriations to Howard as it did to state institutions under the Morrill Land Grant Act of 1890. These funds allowed the university to make major renovations to existing buildings, including eliminating fire and safety hazards, as well as to construct new classroom buildings, dormitories, and athletic facilities. The larger operating budget also allowed the university to employ Cornely and Ferebee as campus physicians to men and women, respectively.[67]

According to Cornely, while using local hospitals might seem to be the "logical solution" to student health issues, such arrangements in fact did not address students' special needs. Hospitals such as Freedmen's "all to often have a tendency to stress treatment and care rather than prevention, health education and the promotion of good health habits," which Cornely felt were the primary missions of a college health service.[68]

This metaphor of health service as home proved immensely popular among students and parents. Colleges and universities that lacked independent student health services found themselves out of step with their competitors and quickly moved to upgrade their facilities. Dartmouth College lagged behind the other Ivy League institutions in that it did not provide a health service for specifically for students. Instead, students sought care at Hanover's Mary Hitchcock Memorial Hospital. Students with contagious diseases, such as measles, mumps, and chicken pox, were removed from their dormitory rooms and sent to the "pest house" (an isolation hospital on the edge of town), where they would not infect other students. The attendants invited students to write in the hospital's log books, where they routinely mocked the quality of the food, beds, and staff. Some students enjoyed the opportunity to escape the pressures of academic life and get a "good rest" at the "pest house in the sticks." Others complained about the conditions of the "Hanover prison," where they were the victims of "hard hearts, and harder beds, phantoms and other insectivore, not to mention bloody noses and slimy baths of mercury." When the isolation hospital was full, as it often was when epidemics of measles and mumps swept through the student residences, inmates enjoyed a "gay social life," playing cards and cribbage with fellow residents. One patient suggested that the quarters could be improved by installing a pool table and cabaret show and staffing the wards with attendants "chosen from a Ziegfield [*sic*] chorus." Parents, conversely, became increasingly dissatisfied with the lack of supervision at the pest house, where students were cared for by medical school students who routinely smuggled alcohol and cigarettes to their charges.[69]

In 1925, Edward Kimball Hall and Sally Hall donated funds to the college for a student infirmary in memory of their son, Dick, who had died of polio the previous year. The Halls hoped that Dick's House would "provide a home for students of the College when they are sick, either in mind or body, and need a bit of home life and home care." The Halls had visited other college infirmaries and hoped to give Dartmouth a facility meeting the standards set by other members of the Ivy League while providing the "atmosphere of a gracious home and the unmistakable imprint of Dartmouth." President Ernest Martin Hopkins wrote to the Halls that he had "been worried and often panic-stricken when one of our boys has been sick. Lately with the Hospital crowded to its doors, as its reputation has increased, I have not seen our way out if illness broke out in any number of cases among the boys. And always I have wanted better quarters for the individual boy than usually were available." Hopkins was certain that the new Dick's House would be the "next best thing to going to their own homes when they are in need of either the care or the surroundings that the dormitory or fraternity house is unable to furnish." Yet students and parents still had to pay for services at Dick's House. A 1936 survey indicated that a "majority of students failed to seek medical help in event of illness because of reluctance to incur out-of-pocket expenses for professional advice and care." This prompted Dartmouth to follow the lead of other institutions of higher education and create a prepaid comprehensive health service.[70]

Despite ongoing reports about the importance of health services, particularly for students of limited means, college administrators remained reluctant to increase the portion of the budget spent on health services and to guarantee positions for college physicians. The financial problems that many colleges and universities experienced during the Great Depression threatened further to reduce the budget for college health. College administrators who wanted to save money frequently targeted college health centers for budget cuts, since officials believed these facilities duplicated services available in the surrounding community. Even physicians at historically black institutions, where there was a dearth of health care alternatives in the surrounding community, found themselves having to defend their work. According to Ferebee, the board of directors and some of the instructors of Howard University really "were not terribly impressed with the needs of the Health Service. They didn't know what it meant."[71]

The AMA remained opposed to college health services as well, even though only 10 percent of all colleges and universities in the country had health services and only 7 percent of all those aged between eighteen and twenty-four attended college during this time.[72] As a challenge to the CCMC's work, the AMA started its Bureau of Medical Economics to study the costs of health care delivery. The bureau's earliest reports included a scathing critique of college and university student health services. Although the bureau supported the preventive services offered by colleges and universities, such as annual physical examinations, hygiene instruction, physical education, vaccinations, and sanitary supervision of the campus environment, the AMA opposed having college health centers provide medical care for students, particularly if such services could be provided by doctors in the area.[73] Faced with continuing opposition from the mainstream medical profession, college physicians looked for additional ways to justify their work. Linking the health of student bodies to the health of the nation would be a major strategy in this endeavor.

CHAPTER 5

Selling Hygiene

In 1927, Stanford University Press issued a report, *The Status of Hygiene Programs in Institutions of Higher Education in the United States*, as part of its University Series in the Medical Sciences. Authored by Thomas A. Storey, Stanford's director of hygiene and physical education for men, the report was a project of the Presidents' Committee of Fifty on College Hygiene, which was organized in 1922 as a result of the joint support of the U.S. Interdepartmental Social Hygiene Board and the American Social Hygiene Association. The Committee of Fifty's stated aim was to study the status of college health departments in the United States and increase support for these programs. Given the affiliations with social hygiene organizations, concerns about the spread of venereal disease during World War I were at the forefront of the committee's work. In 1918, the Sixty-fifth Congress passed the Chamberlain-Kahn Act, which created the Venereal Disease Division of the U.S. Public Health Service and the U.S. International Social Hygiene Board (ISHB). Storey, then head of the Hygiene Department at City College of New York, was appointed as the ISHB's executive secretary in charge of dispersing the $4 million in funds appropriated to the board. Included in this appropriation was the sum of $300,000 annually for two years be paid to forty normal schools, colleges, and universities, including two "colored" institutions, that the ISHB believed qualified to discover and develop more effective educational programs to prevent venereal disease. Institutions receiving these funds had to agree to provide matching funds at least equal to those provided by the board as well as make the hygiene department a permanent part of the institution. The board chose to target college and university students partly because of their age and maturity but also because the college program "would lead to permanency of education influence" by increasing the "number of informed, self-respecting, and self-reliant persons, who as teachers, parents, and community leaders will exert influence in the schools, in the family, and in every educational agency in society."[1] Although funds were intended mainly for educational measures to prevent venereal disease, these resources also allowed the selected normal schools, colleges, and universities to expand health services for both male and female students. In addition to instructing students in "moral prophylaxis," these hygiene departments instituted a wide range of medical services, including emergency care, inoculations for contagious diseases, laboratory tests, and regular medical checkups.[2]

By the middle part of the decade, the American Medical Association (AMA) had launched a campaign against federally funded health programs.[3] Student health services also came under attack, as did funding provided by the ISHB. The AMA condemned the board as another form of "state medicine" that had invaded the territory of the medical profession. Consequently, total appropriations for the ISHB fell to just $60,000 in 1926.[4]

To counter this opposition from the AMA, Storey described the "strategic public educational opportunities" of college hygiene programs. While only 6.69 percent of all persons in the United States aged twenty-one or older had graduated from college, "slightly more than half of the positions of great influence in this country were reported as filled by men and women who had been students in or received degrees from institutions of college rank." Storey concluded that college hygiene programs not only improved the health of the individual student but also helped "sell hygiene" to the larger society by convincing future leaders to adopt the most up-to-date laws of public health and personal hygiene. These students, so educated, would go on to shape the "health standards, the health investments, and the health practices of the public."[5]

This notion of "selling hygiene" to the American public via its most educated citizens formed part of a larger strategy to make college health programs acceptable to the mainstream medical profession. College physicians argued that by virtue of their training as allopathic physicians, they could help contribute to the growing cultural authority of allopathic medicine.[6] According to John Sundwall, colleges and universities commonly appointed as directors of health departments "successful football coach[es]" who were "ignorant of the sciences and interests which make up modern medicine and hygiene" and supported a variety of health "fads" such as Fletcherism, vegetarianism, and hydrotherapy.[7] Sundwall and other college physicians argued that college health programs could help elevate allopathic medicine in the public mind by stamping out "quackery" and "superstition" once and for all. By "selling hygiene" to students through regular physical examinations and doctor visits, Storey and other college health professionals argued that they were "selling" the reputation of the medical profession those who would go on to shape the health of the nation as a whole.

A key focus of college health work in the 1910s and 1920s were the health dangers posed by the "revolution in manners and morals" on college campuses during this time.[8] On the eve of World War I, student sexual practices were radically changing. Dr. Max J. Exner, public health officer for the Young Men's Christian Association (YMCA), reported that more than half of his sample of 948 college men had engaged in sexual practices of some kind. More than 60 percent had practiced "self-abuse," 17 percent had also engaged in intercourse, and 2 percent described engaging in "various perverted practices," which Exner did not specify. Studies of the sex behavior of female college graduates conducted by Stanford's Clelia Duel Mosher and by New York City correction commissioner Katherine Bement Davis in the 1910s and 1920s indicated that similar changes were occurring on a smaller scale among female undergraduates.[9] Reformers had long been concerned about "declining morals" among working-class, immigrant youth. The fact that "respectable" college and university students also engaged in such "radical" sexual practices disturbed many parents, health professionals, and officials in higher education.

At historically black colleges, particularly those sponsored by religious denominations, undergraduates were also rebelling against paternalistic policies aimed at preserving their health and respectability. Students demanded an end to compulsory chapel attendance, dress codes, mandatory physical education, and strict rules regulating social interaction between male and female students. Like their white counterparts, middle-class black undergraduates wanted "the ability to control their own bodies, the freedom to consume and experience bodily pleasure without fear of being punished."[10]

Black physicians and educators found these trends especially disturbing because their students encountered the same racial stereotypes about black health and sexuality as did lower-class African Americans. To combat white prejudice, black reformers explicitly linked racial health and middle-class standards of sexual respectability. African American leaders targeted students at normal schools and colleges in the belief that they would disseminate high moral standards and hygiene information to the race more generally. Noted black activist and clubwoman Mary Church Terrell, for example, told students at Howard that "blacks could not afford to abandon traditional morality even if many young whites were doing so."[11]

These changes in student behavior were alarming, given the growing incidence of venereal disease. The Wasserman test for syphilis became a routine part of most college entrance physical examinations. The infection rate among college students was found to be very low (less than 1 percent, compared with 5–10 percent in the general population) and was frequently attributed to congenital transmission, casual contact, and other "innocent" forms of infection. Yet the fact that any cases at all occurred among the most privileged section of the population played into larger fears about racial degeneration. To address these concerns, college health programs created new initiatives to improve disease prevention and treatment for young people.

As Go the Colleges So Goes the Nation

The term *social hygiene* represented both a euphemism for the control of what were then called venereal diseases as well as a new approach to prevention of these afflictions. Social hygiene differed from earlier "purity crusades," which shielded young people from moral and physical dangers via a "conspiracy of silence" about sexual matters. Social hygienists attacked the sexual double standard, supporting total abstinence before marriage for both men and women. Yet social hygienists believed that education rather than scare tactics constituted the best way to protect the health of the nation's youth.[12]

The social hygiene movement also had a broad vision of its preventive work that went beyond simply stamping out venereal disease. The American Social Hygiene Association (ASHA) was founded in 1914 "on the sound theory that any influence that works for the improvement of hygiene in general must work for the improvement of social hygiene."[13] The organization's first president, Harvard's president emeritus, Charles W. Eliot, declared that social hygiene should incorporate all aspects of the social environment affecting students. He therefore advocated bodily exercise, moderation in eating, and abstinence from tobacco, alcohol, hot spices, and "all other drugs which impair self-control, even momentarily" as essential to the movement's goals.[14]

The social hygiene movement was strongly influenced by the ideas of

Sigmund Freud and G. Stanley Hall, who emphasized that sexual impulses were normal parts of both male and female adolescent development. According to Hall, psychoanalysis demonstrated how the sex instinct pervaded "every sphere of life, even those in which it was not suspected." The challenge for educators, Hall concluded, was not to suppress sexuality but "to short-circuit, transmute it, and turn it on to develop the higher powers of man."[15] On the college level, Hall agreed that students "should have the medical truth about sex diseases (not perversions) as plainly, directly and compactly" as possible, but "too much relevance should not be placed on this." Above all "warning methods" should go attempts to divert sexual energy through physical activity, "wholesome religious interest," "literary fervor," and other innocuous activities.[16]

Social hygienists considered the college population central to their efforts, claiming that students who were educated in scientific principles related to sex would pass this information along to others. As Storey put it, normal school students were especially critical to the social hygiene movement because they would go on to shape educational hygiene in the nation's schools. College and university students too would become leaders in public health policy in cities, states, and the nation, thereby raising the standards of public health and private hygiene.[17]

Students proved an eager audience for sex education. At the forefront of student-led endeavors was the Student Department of the International Committee of the YMCA. The Student YMCA's interest in social hygiene constituted part of a larger transition away from the organization's traditional focus on religious piety and individual salvation. Prior to World War I, the intercollegiate YMCAs had served as "healthy alternatives" to fraternities and the "chief temptations of American students"—drinking, smoking, gambling, and above all sexual impurity. By the mid-1910s, however, the Student Department's earlier emphasis on personal evangelism was replaced with interest in social justice and progressive political causes. This movement into the message of the Social Gospel put the student division at odds with the larger YMCA, which roundly condemned the "revolution in manners and morals" among the nation's youth. The student division, in contrast, wanted to harness the rebellious energy of the Jazz Age to create a just society. Embracing the social message of Christ's life and words, the intercollegiate YMCAs sought to use the young people of the era to eliminate such social evils as prostitution, child labor, economic and racial inequality, and international war.[18]

At the same time, the YMCA was responding to broader cultural anxieties about the dangers of single-sex organizations. The rise of a thriving homosexual male subculture in the nation's cities during 1910s and 1920s escalated anxieties about a growing "homosexual menace." This development prompted the YMCA to depart from its earlier focus on programs for men and boys and deliberately to seek the participation of women in the organization's activities as well as partnerships with the Young Women's Christian Association (YWCA). By the 1910s, both the YMCA and YWCA were emulating broader trends in the social interaction between men and women, as popular forms of entertainment and public spaces encouraged the rise of a mixed-sex, or heterosocial, youth culture. Both organizations were also trying to deflect larger concerns that single-sex organizations caused young people to engage in "sexual perversions"—that is, homosexual relationships.[19] To this end, the Student Department of the YMCA invited Exner to begin a program of sex education for college men and women in the 1910s. Exner believed such a program to be "strategic" because it would affect sex education in other fields. "As go the colleges so goes the nation," he declared.[20]

To aid his efforts, Exner requested funding from the Rockefeller Foundation's Bureau of Social Hygiene to study the relevant literature in the field to "standardize it for use by our college leaders" and to train "thoroughly desirable and capable men who may be used as lecturers in the colleges."[21] Exner hoped the YMCA sex education program would "lift the subject more fully out of the grossly physical into the realm of the affections, and thus into a finer atmosphere of appreciation and thinking." Exner added, "The students are hungry for this kind of teaching and their splendid response to it shows that at heart every student is an idealist."[22] YMCA field secretaries reported audiences of more than one thousand at their sex education lectures, with students staying for hours after the speaker concluded to ask additional questions.[23] Exner told John D. Rockefeller that he and other lecturers made a deep impression on both faculty and students, demonstrated "not only by the cordial words of colleges but especially by the large number and the nature of personal interviews following the addresses."[24] Students at black colleges were especially eager to adopt the YMCA's sex education program, since they saw it as a way to overcome white prejudice by keeping the new "manners and morals" of the Jazz Age "within the boundaries of respectability."[25] Consequently, by 1920, 113 African American schools had YMCA chapters, and sex education constituted a significant portion of their activities.[26]

Rockefeller believed that sex education was particularly important for female students because so many young women became teachers. Yet he was also was concerned about preserving sexual propriety, insisting that women should receive instruction in sex education separately from men. Rockefeller complained, "It is difficult to find just the right women physicians who are capable of presenting the subject properly," alleging that many female physicians were too sentimental and lacked the ability to balance the religious and scientific points of view. He was nevertheless convinced that it was more appropriate for young women to receive instruction from female physicians.[27] To assist with these efforts, Exner enlisted Dr. Anna L. Brown of the YWCA's national board to help locate and train women physicians in sex education for female students. By the late 1910s, the board employed fourteen women physicians to assist in their sex education efforts, including such noted college physicians as Mary B. Ritter of the University of California, Berkeley.[28]

The National Interfraternity Conference (NIC) also proved instrumental in establishing social hygiene programs on college campuses. The NIC was formed in 1909, when a group of twenty-six fraternities came together to discuss "pressing issues of the day," not the least of which was growing criticism about the "social dissipation" of fraternity life.[29] In the early 1920s, the NIC formed the Social Hygiene Committee to collaborate with the Exner and other members of the ASHA in conducting a joint study of 202 colleges and universities. They sought to create a standard curriculum in sex education for colleges and universities. The report, issued in 1922, proposed that "appropriate sex content be integrated in the college subjects to which sex has a natural relation," based on "the principle that sex teaching comes most normally as a part of the broader subjects to which it appropriately belongs," such as "biology, psychology, sociology, ethics, physical education and hygiene, the home-making sciences and the teaching of literature." According to Exner, shortly after the report was released, nearly 25 percent of the institutions that participated in the report had adopted various suggestions. He predicted "with confidence that in the next ten years much progress will be made in promoting wholesome and successful personal and social sex adjustment."[30]

Support from private foundations became critical in the 1920s, as the AMA's battle against "socialized medicine" caused the demise of the ISHB. To make up for the drop in federal funding, voluntary organizations and private foundations such as the YMCA, the ASHA, the Interfraternity Council, and the Bureau of Social Hygiene continued to provide funding for college and university sex education programs. To further its college work, the ASHA financed the creation of the Presidents' Committee of Fifty on College Hygiene in 1922, with Eliot as chair and Storey as executive secretary. Other committee members included male and female college presidents from public and private institutions around the country, male and female directors of college health programs, and prominent figures in the field of public health, including William H. Welch, director of the School of Hygiene and Public Health at Johns Hopkins University.[31] Support from ASHA led more than two hundred colleges, universities, and normal schools to appoint social hygiene committees, which prepared materials aimed at integrating social hygiene into existing courses in biology, psychology, sociology, physiology, hygiene, education, physical education, and home economics. By the early 1930s, noted one ASHA report, 111 colleges had some form of social hygiene material in their curriculum.[32]

Although the age of the student population made college sex education programs less controversial than those for younger groups, some faculty and administrators objected despite widespread student support. Undergraduates at Northwestern, for example, declared in 1925 that "the faculty is old and fogeyish, and that sex hygiene is not given sufficient prominence."[33] A formidable opponent was Harvard psychologist Hugo Muensterberg, who vigorously condemned the country's declining moral standards in his regular column in the *New York Times.* Although Muensterberg's chief targets were Broadway and Hollywood, he also complained that the "lack of discipline in education" posed as much a "threat to the social safety" as did smutty literature, theater, and film. "What can be more fraught with dangers," Muensterberg asked, "than to abolish the policy of silence and to uphold the policy of talking and talking about sexual matters with those whose minds were still untouched by the lure." Muensterberg condemned Eliot's work with the ASHA, calling his and other reformers' attempts at sex education ineffective and inappropriate. Instead, Muensterberg believed, the "old-fashioned policy of silence" was the best way to curb the sexual appetites of the young.[34]

Even comparatively liberal physicians, such as Mosher, who had conducted a frank survey of the sexual practices of her adult female patients in the 1890s and early 1900s, despaired privately about the challenges of reigning in the exuberant young coeds of the Jazz Age. In a 1926 diary entry, Mosher wrote, "My Victorian sense of decent reticence is constantly shocked" by the questions and behavior of her students. Although she believed "these girls should have any question they asked answered honestly and sanely," she was mortified about what "they should be able to ask without hesitation in class." She declared wistfully, "It is a new age, new thinking, new ideals, or does it mean no ideals?"[35] To alleviate qualms about their work, supporters of college social hygiene programs explicitly linked the safety of student bodies and the viability of the nation's body politic.

Social Hygiene and Human Betterment

Although college students made up a small percentage of the young adult population throughout the twentieth century, college physicians argued that protecting elite student bodies from physical and moral dangers was essential to "race betterment" among the better social classes. In this sense, college hygiene programs overlapped with the broader eugenics movement of the early twentieth century.[36] In general, social hygienists on the college level embraced a broad vision of eugenics that included aspects of genetic determinism and environmentalism. College officials argued that selective breeding could be used to improve human society and supported sterilization of the "unfit," restrictions on immigration by members of "undesirable" ethnic groups, and other eugenic measures aimed at weeding out those of "inferior blood." Within this viewpoint, college students were superior to other young adults and therefore should be protected and encouraged to reproduce. Reports about the declining birthrate among the college-educated population were discouraging in this regard. According to Metropolitan Life Insurance statistician Louis I. Dublin, while college-educated individuals lived longer and their children were healthier, college graduates—particularly alumnae of women's colleges—had fewer children than those from the less educated, predominantly immigrant classes. Dublin warned that the "race stock which laid the foundations of our institutions during the critical period of our national existence is in larger areas no longer maintaining itself and its place is being taken gradually but surely by foreign races, which, as we have seen, are reproducing rapidly."[37]

During the 1910s, elite colleges such as Harvard, Columbia, Cornell, Brown, and Northwestern began disseminating information on eugenics in courses on biology, sociology, and psychology. The state land-grant universities also played a prominent role in the popularization of eugenics by instituting the country life movement, which focused on enhancing the health and reproductive potential of white, native-born rural inhabitants. The country life movement promoted eugenics through rural schools, county extension services in agriculture and home economics, "better baby" and "fitter family" contests at state fairs, and college courses in biology and genetics. These programs were especially popular in the Southeast, where eugenics reinforced the region's system of white supremacy. College physicians alleged that frequent inbreeding had led to a high incidence of hereditary disorders and congenital disorders in white students from the rural South. Like other medical professionals who worked on what were conceived as distinctively southern health problems, college physicians hoped to contribute to the regeneration of white racial stock by eliminating the causes of ill health in white southerners. By the late 1920s, more than three hundred colleges and universities offered courses that covered eugenic themes, with as many as twenty thousand students enrolled.[38]

Yet, college social hygienists also supported euthenics, or the notion that American racial stock in general could be improved through better nutrition, health care, and other preventive health measures. According to Storey, "The health of the student depends not only on his heritage but also upon the living functional experience of that heritage with that environment."[39] To illustrate this point, college hygiene departments published data from mandatory physical examinations. These reports argued that survival of the fittest individuals, combined with advances in public health and preventive medicine, resulted in drastic improvements in the bodies of American college students. Dudley Allen Sargent, for example, wrote in 1914 that his "long experience and careful observation" of students at Harvard and Radcliffe "have shown us that physical education, in its best and broadest sense, is one of the most important factors in the betterment of the race." Exercise was especially important for women, since the development of strong pelvic muscles would lead to the birth of healthier children. Thus, individual physical improvement led to a "better race of children, so that we may consider physical education an agent in our modern sciences of euthenics and eugenics."[40]

Physicians made a similar case for other forms of hygiene instruction, such as proper habits of diet, dress, and rest. Again, women students constituted a central part of this mission. Dr. Carolyn Geisel, physician at Shorter Women's College in Rome, Georgia, wrote that the first aim of a hygiene department was "to build a strong body for the student herself" so that she would become "a balanced, strong unit in the support of this liberty-loving government of ours." The second and equally important aim was "to give the student such complete knowledge of Health and Homemaking as will secure strong bodies to her family."[41]

According to Sundwall, education in euthenics was just as important for male students. "College students, by virtue of their educational opportunities, should become and usually do become leaders in matters pertaining to human betterment," he argued. Consequently, college hygiene departments should be headed by medical doctors well trained in all the scientific principles of health promotion, not just physical exercise, to pass along to students knowledge of modern public health.[42]

College health professionals believed that hygiene education was especially important for rural areas in the southeastern states, which many considered desperately in need of modern public health reforms. Emblematic of the South's backwardness in sanitation was the parasite hookworm, which thrived in feces-contaminated soil and was easily transmitted by walking barefoot through infected areas. The parasite eventually lodged in the lining of the victim's small intestine, where it drew on the host's blood and caused severe iron-deficiency anemia, especially in individuals who were already malnourished. White southern college students who flocked to state universities, medical schools, and tuition-free agricultural colleges constituted one of the first populations examined for hookworm after 1900 and, like impoverished whites and African Americans of all classes, demonstrated a high incidence of the disease.[43] The ubiquitous presence of hookworm in the South regardless of race or social status prompted an aggressive antihookworm campaign by the Rockefeller Foundation's Sanitary Commission starting in 1909. To counter locals' objections that the antihookworm campaign was a "Yankee plot" to deride the South and sell shoes to its inhabitants, the Sanitary Commission enlisted the cooperation of regional public health officials and educators. Sanitary inspectors targeted their programs at college students, believing that taking advantage of a "snob factor" would help make the campaign more acceptable among the population at large. In the words of John Ferrell of the North Carolina state public health service, by making hookworm testing "fashionable" among the "better class of people[,] the most highly infected class will be more easily reached and will seek examination." These students would then go back to their communities and would by virtue of their social standing "prove to be unconscious workers for the cause during the summer."[44] Despite this campaign, in the mid-1930s, University of North Carolina head physician W. Reece Berryhill reported "*mirabile dictu* in this enlightened age six cases of hookworm."[45]

African American physicians and educators, who were equally concerned about the inadequacy of health care and preventive medicine available to black college students, also adopted some aspects of eugenic thinking. Civil rights pioneer W. E. B. Du Bois, for example, observed that the black middle class was beginning to breed "for brains, for efficiency, and for beauty" and that the products of these endeavors were "beginning to appear in the colleges of the North in appreciable numbers."[46] Dublin observed, "Race suicide among the higher classes of negroes is present in as true a sense among the middle classes of whites."[47] African American reformers argued that race progress hinged on eradicating venereal disease and prostitution, encouraging the production and survival of "well-born" children, and cultivating high moral standards in young men and women. College-educated clubwomen sponsored "better baby" contests for black children and founded a national "Department of Eugenics" with the goal of spreading the "gospel of clean manhood and womanhood" among the black community through sex education and home economics classes in schools, colleges, and county extension programs.[48] Like their counterparts at white institutions, physicians at black colleges and universities believed that social hygiene for undergraduates was essential to improving the health of the race as a whole.

National Negro Health Week and Natural Leaders

Booker T. Washington was among the first African American educators to recognize the importance of hygiene education to the larger cause of racial uplift. In 1915, Washington enlisted the support of Howard University, the National Medical Association, the National Insurance Association, and the National Negro Business League in starting National Negro Health Week at Tuskegee Institute. The new organization sought "to raise consciousness of proper health care" among African Americans.[49] Tuskegee, Howard, and other black colleges and universities served as focal points for various Negro Health Week events such as essay contests, student presentations, and exhibits. Voluntary health organizations such as the ASHA and the National Tuberculosis Association (NTA) were especially eager to cultivate the support of black college physicians as well as black fraternities, sororities, and other student organizations.[50] As Dr. Walter Clarke, executive director of the ASHA, observed in 1943, the organization deliberately sought to enlist "natural leaders" at Negro colleges to assist in combating the scourges of syphilis and gonorrhea.[51]

These "natural leaders" included Paul B. Cornely and Dorothy Ferebee at the Howard University Health Services. Both physicians embodied the "southern missionary work" undertaken by black physicians raised and/or educated in the North during the early twentieth century. Because of their connections with white public health organizations and medical institutions in the North, these "medical missionaries" were better able than southern black doctors to gain recognition from the white establishment of the significance of black health problems. As ambassadors from the North, they were also in a better position to initiate discussions between black and white health professionals on the best ways to solve Negro health problems.[52]

Cornely argued that health education was especially urgent at Negro colleges, since the most pronounced differences in mortality between blacks and whites were "found in the ages between 15 and 25 years. At this level," Cornely observed, "the death rate for colored boys and young men is nearly two and a half times that for whites, and the rate among colored girls is more than three times that for young white women." While much of this discrepancy could be attributed to "dire need for facilities and sufficient competent health personnel to give adequate services to Negroes," Cornely also argued that the "prevalence of superstitions, poor health habits, improper attitudes, and warped ideas about health are unfavorable to the health status of this section of the population." The solution, Cornely argued, was the "proper nurture in health education" of college men and women, which "should produce leaders with the proper health perspective, ideals, attitudes, and visions, who will be able to formulate, mould, and direct public opinion on health matters." The accomplishment of other major health goals, including better health services and improvement of standards of living, depended heavily on reaching the college student population.[53]

One of the best examples of the use of college students to improve the health of the black community was the Mississippi Health Project, a series of health clinics for rural sharecroppers in the Mississippi Delta organized by volunteers from Howard University's Alpha Kappa Alpha (AKA), the oldest black sorority in the nation, and led by Ferebee. The Mississippi Health Project was an attempt by black middle-class women to bridge the gap between themselves and the less fortunate by serving as "health missionaries" to the black poor. Although the AKA members also faced racial discrimination, their education and economic status were markedly better than the mostly illiterate, impoverished sharecroppers they served.[54] Nevertheless, the economic circumstances of the AKA women and other Howard students did not mean that they enjoyed the same health status as did white undergraduates. Ferebee remembered that "when Dr. Cornely induced me—not induced, but persuaded me—to come to the Health Service, I was just finishing my internships and doing community work in Washington. He said, 'You remain at Howard University. I think you will find here almost as many needs as those that you talk about for Mississippi.'"[55]

Philanthropic organizations, most notably the Rockefeller Foundation's General Education Board (GEB), played a major role in these efforts to improve public health at black institutions. Although frequently derided for kowtowing to the bigotry of the white South, by the 1930s even its harshest critic, Du Bois, grudgingly admitted the GEB was atoning for its past mistakes. Given the "lamentable failure of democracy in the South," Du Bois wrote in the *Crisis* in 1930, "the General Education Board in later years has been the salvation of education among Negroes."[56] Wary of offending the white establishment, the GEB equally distributed its funds to black and white institutions. In the case of black education, the GEB gave funds to state agencies for Negro education, all of which were directed by whites, albeit comparatively liberal ones who believed in opening educational opportunities to African Americans. As the title implied, the major goal of the GEB's New Southern Program was to improve general education in southern institutions, but given the Rockefellers' interest in promoting science and medicine, health education played a significant role in the board's agenda. According to 1940 GEB survey, health education and health services for black students were totally inadequate, even in the comparatively progressive state of North Carolina, where white leaders were more committed to advancing black health and education than most of the region's whites. Believing that health education would be futile unless students had access to adequate health care, the GEB helped fund comprehensive health services at several southern black colleges.[57]

Cornely was aware of the dilemmas posed by preventive efforts singling out blacks for special attention. On the one hand, he agreed with such efforts, stating that nothing could be timelier than social hygiene education among Negroes.[58] On the other hand, he recognized that such programs had the potential to reinforce white stereotypes about black sexuality, which characterized African Americans as a "notoriously syphilis-soaked race."[59] As one ASHA member told Clarke after a presentation before a group of African American physicians in New Jersey, "Many of the physicians in the audience were unanimous in their opinion, that programs directed especially along these lines were obnoxious to the negroes in general, because they created the inference that the negro race was composed chiefly of diseased individuals who were potentially dangerous to others."[60] Thus, while Cornely believed that "special charts, literature, and motion pictures must be developed if we are going to make any progress in this field," he warned that development of these materials "should be done with a great deal of care." Above all, Cornely insisted, educational efforts had to be undertaken by black physicians and nurses, who could more effectively serve as liaisons between white-dominated voluntary organizations and the African American community.[61]

Hoping to defuse controversies over hygiene programs that focused undue attention on the consequences of sexual behavior, physicians in both white and black institutions turned to another plague that disproportionately affected the college-aged population: tuberculosis. During the 1910s and 1920s, physicians in college health centers gradually realized that routine exclusion of those with noticeably active cases of tuberculosis not only constituted an inadequate measure to combat the disease but also led to wastage of students who had the potential to succeed academically. The antituberculosis campaign, like the social hygiene movement before it, represented an attempt to salvage and rehabilitate diseased student bodies.

A Dangerous Age

Despite attempts to exclude tubercular students from admission, tuberculosis remained a major health threat for college students in the 1920s and 1930s. The routine use of tuberculin tests in college entrance physicals, which began in the early 1920s, led to the discovery of large numbers of "pretubercular" college students—that is, those who tested positive on the tuberculin test but did not have active cases of the disease. The infection rate was as high as 50 or 60 percent among all undergraduates in the northeastern United States and 80 percent among students in the Southwest. Infection rates were even higher in medical and nursing students, with some schools reporting that it was not unusual for the entire graduating class to test positive for tuberculosis.[62] These statistics were especially disturbing since tuberculosis among the population at large was declining and because tuberculosis was a disease usually associated with poverty.[63] The discovery of high infection rates among American college students, regardless of race, class, or gender, was alarming for several reasons. First, although advances in microbiology had demonstrated that TB was not an inherited disease, the eugenics movement had popularized the belief that susceptibility to TB infection was a sure sign of genetic inferiority. Tuberculosis, along with venereal disease, remained on the "list of disorders whose carriers could not legally marry under laws usually labeled 'eugenic.'" Some states even recommended sterilization of women with tuberculosis, primarily to protect women's health but also prevent transmission of the disease to children.[64]

Therefore, TB still carried with it a powerful social stigma. In fact, some colleges reported difficulty in getting students to comply with testing precisely because of fears that a positive reaction would lead to social ostracism and dismissal from college. Esmond R. Long, for example, noted that the high compliance rate at the University of Pennsylvania owed much to a "dean who runs the test with a mixture of genial cajolery and ferocious threats that is extraordinarily effective."[65] Treatment options for those who developed the disease were limited in the era before antibiotics. Although new surgical techniques such as artificial pneumothorax and thoracoplasty had been developed, confinement to a sanitarium was still the major therapy for those with tuberculosis. Yet recovery rates for patients admitted to these facilities were poor, and sanatoria lacked enough space to accommodate all those who needed treatment.[66] Epidemiological data indicated that the years from fifteen to twenty-five were an especially "dangerous age" for those who tested positive for the disease, with death rates more than six times higher than those for either children or older adults. According to a pamphlet published by the NTA in 1927, tuberculosis presented a "peculiar danger" for those in the first decade of maturity, when "the sparks of latent disease may be fanned into the flame of the adult type of tuberculosis." Although the death rate had fallen significantly among the population as a whole, according to the NTA, it remained the chief cause of death for those in their late teens and early twenties. The death rate was especially high in young women—about one-third greater than in young men of the same age. Medical experts attributed this high mortality rate to young people's "carelessness" about their health as well as their tendency to "overwork and overplay," all of which increased the chance that the "seed" of tuberculosis would take root and reach its full "harvest."[67]

Concerns about the high rate of tuberculosis infection in college students created both challenges and possibilities for those involved in college health. One of the virtues of using tuberculosis as a tool to sell college health work was that it avoided some of the negative overtones associated with earlier social hygiene programs. College physicians hoped that because tuberculosis was a less volatile subject and the incidence of the disease was much greater, the threat of this disease could more easily justify increased expenditures for college health.

Nevertheless, the antituberculosis campaign for college students, like tuberculosis prevention work more generally, borrowed much of its imagery from the social hygiene movement. Lee H. Ferguson of Case Western Reserve University in Cleveland, for example, claimed that "lack of parental supervision and overabundance of social life" were the major factors in the surprisingly high incidence of tuberculosis in college students.[68] Physicians were especially critical of changing gender roles, blaming the greater prevalence of tuberculosis in college women on flappers, who "embarked upon a career of wholesale smashing of conservative ideals of feminine behavior." These critics argued that young women who refused to wear sensible clothing, who dieted excessively in pursuit of boyish figures, who smoked cigarettes, or who otherwise abandoned traditional standards of feminine decorum were at greater risk for contracting tuberculosis.[69] Other tuberculosis articles offered a more sympathetic view of female college students but still blamed high infection rates on young women's unwise choices in running their personal lives. Physicians complained about young women who, freed from parental supervision for the first time, failed to get enough sleep or spent their limited funds on cosmetics, beauty treatments, fancy clothes, and entertainment rather than on nourishing food and sensible attire.[70]

Tuberculosis literature suggested that the reckless antics of young men also put them at great risk for the disease. Esmond Long and Florence Seibert of the Phipps Institute, for example, argued that while mortality from tuberculosis was higher in women, male students were "less restricted in their contacts outside the home and therefore have a greater opportunity for chance infection."[71] Campus life further encouraged the spread of tuberculosis among college men. Male undergraduates tended to be "happy-go-lucky" about their health and would not seek the advice of a physician until the disease was well advanced, Long observed. Thus, rather than wait for students to come to the doctor, "the physician must go to him. This may appear to violate some of the fundamental principles of our age-old concepts of the physician-patient relationship," Long acknowledged, "but times are changing rapidly in this and other respects, and the tuberculosis will not wait until the ethics of the situation are properly settled."[72]

Articles on college prevention programs also drew on eugenic concepts, particularly the belief that areas with higher concentrations of immigrants were more dangerous than other regions of the country. For example, in a comparison of screening programs at various institutions, Charles E. Shepard of Stanford University observed that positive reactors were "more frequent in colleges that draw students from densely populated districts, such as the University of Pennsylvania and Yale University, than in colleges drawing from chiefly rural districts." Shepard also reported large differences in infection rates between rural and urban areas of the same state. Long and Seibert made similar observations, noting that a significant number of those with active tuberculosis were Jewish students in the professional schools of medicine, law, and business. Although they avoided blaming tuberculosis infection on Jews, the dangers of urban living clearly were a particular cause of concern. However, these reports also argued that no one, regardless of class or ethnicity, was immune from the disease and advocated mass screening of all students to detect cases of tuberculosis before they posed a threat to other students.[73]

The desire to use tuberculosis control as a method of racial improvement was also apparent in the programs started at historically black colleges during the 1920s and 1930s. Tuberculosis prevention in black colleges grew out the NTA's Committee on Tuberculosis among Negroes, whose major goal was to overturn the "attitude all too prevalent that tuberculosis in the Negro is invariably fatal." Rather, they argued, tuberculosis in blacks could be fought with health education. "Knowledge is power," announced one committee report. Unless knowledge of the cause, prevention, and cure of tuberculosis was widely disseminated, the report concluded, "other control measures will be ineffective." The committee members believed that the "most important group to be reached in a health education program for Negroes is the group of Negro students now enrolled in universities, colleges, and teacher training schools." Drawing on Du Bois's notion of the "Talented Tenth" and their role in racial uplift, the committee argued that since nearly 90 percent of these students would become leaders of the Negro race, "any knowledge of health which we can give them would in the course of a few years be multiplied a hundredfold." In addition to mandatory testing of black students, the committee sponsored essay contests, funded research on the incidence of tuberculosis in this group, and helped secure funding for the development of student health activities in black colleges. The committee also attempted to compensate for the racism of the ACHA, which while sympathetic to the problem of tuberculosis in blacks refused to admit black physicians or nurses. This discriminatory policy led to the formation of the National Negro Student Health Association, which worked closely with the NTA Committee on Tuberculosis among Negroes, the Julius Rosenwald Fund, the Phelps Stokes Fund, and other philanthropic organizations to study and prevent the spread of tuberculosis among African Americans.[74]

Surveys of college hygiene programs found vast disparities in the kinds of prevention and treatment programs available to students around the country. At one end of the spectrum were institutions that had part-time nurses who treated emergencies and minor illnesses. At the opposite extreme were large, well-equipped centers with a full-time staff of physicians, surgeons, dentists, and special consultants. These results forced Storey to conclude that the "vast majority" of institutions were not providing adequate care and instruction in hygiene to students "who pass through them on their way to responsible citizenship."[75]

These findings prompted the NTA to fund a national conference on health problems in colleges as a way of developing minimum standards for college and university health programs. Held at Syracuse University in 1931 in conjunction with the ACHA's annual meeting, the conference covered a wide variety of health problems common to college students, but tuberculosis played a major role in the proceedings. The conference's Subcommittee on Tuberculosis recommended that all institutions of higher education create tuberculosis prevention programs. In striking contrast to earlier policies, subcommittee members argued that a diagnosis of tuberculosis did not necessarily mandate exclusion from college. Although they advised that those with severe active cases be dismissed until their conditions improved, those with arrested cases could remain as long as their habits and health status were closely followed by medical personnel. The subcommittee also recommended that institutions of higher education emulate broader national trends in TB prevention and help halt the spread of TB not only through screening programs but also by requiring courses in hygiene and by exerting greater control over the lives of all students. The subcommittee's recommendations included requiring both men and women to live on campus; closely monitoring the sleep, eating, and study habits of students; and mandating physical education for all four years of study.[76]

To implement these recommendations, the ACHA asked the Subcommittee on Tuberculosis to institute a five-year program to expand tuberculosis prevention programs around the country. Working closely with both the NTA and local tuberculosis organizations, the subcommittee helped create tuberculosis screening and prevention programs at institutions that did not have them and worked to enhance existing programs.[77] Subcommittee members hoped that such programs would not only control the spread of tuberculosis but eradicate it from the student body altogether. Through such work, wrote Ferguson, the subcommittee's chair, it would eventually "be considered a disgrace for any college and university to permit one of its students to break down with tuberculosis." He called on all university health personnel to "do our part to strike the shackles of an insidious and treacherous disease from the lives of those entrusted to our care. Then and only then can we count our task as well done."[78]

Supervising female students proved to be simple, since most institutions already had the necessary rules and facilities in place. However, both the NTA and the ACHA recognized the difficulty in increasing regulation of male student life. The groups therefore legitimized their efforts by emphasizing the special threats tuberculosis posed to college men. Articles written by members of the ACHA's Subcommittee on Tuberculosis depicted male students as a strategic natural resource and drew on metaphors of "wasted manpower" to describe TB's toll on college men. Preserving the health of college men became especially critical during the Great Depression, since bad health was closely linked with poverty and dependency. "A college education represents considerable investment of money and educational resources," wrote Shepard. Contraction of tuberculosis caused "serious economic losses to the individual, to the college, and to the community."[79]

Physicians also stressed how tuberculosis affected masculine role identity, drawing on Alfred Adler's work on the inferiority complex to underscore further the necessity of preventive efforts.[80] College health officials argued that male students with advanced tuberculosis frequently had no choice but to withdraw from their studies, thereby limiting their career opportunities and assumption of the male breadwinner role. Physicians argued that the ravages of TB gave young men effeminate, pigeon-chested bodies that exposed sufferers to ridicule by their more "manly" classmates. TB further threatened masculinity by preventing young men from engaging in athletic activities crucial to their acceptance by male peers and to popularity with coeds.[81]

Concerns about military preparedness also played a role in physicians' interest in preventing tuberculosis in college men. During World War I, 12 percent of the 178,000 discharges for disability resulted from active cases of tuberculosis, and TB sufferers made up a sizable percentage of those receiving care in veterans' hospitals. The tuberculosis problem among veterans was so great that during the 1920s, the Veterans' Bureau set up a network of hospitals dedicated solely to the care of tuberculosis. Physicians worried that the problem would be just as severe as the nation prepared for war in the late 1930s and warned that if nothing was done, the U.S. military's fighting strength would be permanently diminished.[82] These fears appeared to be confirmed by statistics collected by the Senate's Wartime Subcommittee on Health and Education, which found that more than 4.5 million men were found unfit for duty because of physical or mental defects. According to the Senate's 1945 report, the high incidence of tuberculosis, venereal disease, and other preventable diseases and disorders represented a "serious drain" on U.S. manpower.[83]

The efforts to "sell hygiene" by appealing to U.S. manpower needs increased support for college health programs in the decades following World War II. Surveys indicated that the number of colleges with health services increased from 10 percent in the early 1920s to more than 60 percent by the mid-1950s and that funding for college health programs in general increased substantially during this period.[84] The findings of President Harry S. Truman's Commission on Higher Education lent further support to the importance of college health programs. In a 1947 report, the commission stated that one of the major goals of higher education was to help the individual student "improve and maintain his own health and to cooperate actively and intelligently in solving community health problems." The report argued that "in any society[,] human resources are of paramount importance, and when the physical health and vitality of any large proportion of the people are less than they might be, these resources are seriously impaired." The report found colleges and universities in the United States "doing far less than they might to dispel the ignorance that lies at the root of the ill health of many of our people." The commission members concluded by noting the need for a major reorientation of college health programs and by recommending that instruction in health matters and care of the physical health of the student body be centralized in one department headed by a medical professional.[85]

By the mid-1950s, physicians had convinced most administrators that "while educational institutions were not health centers, it was the duty of the college or university to provide an environment that is conducive to intellectual pursuits." If students as well as faculty and staff were "not protected from preventable health hazards," observed one college president at the Fourth National Conference for Health in Colleges in 1954, "the college is not discharging its educational responsibility."[86]

At the same time, the spread of group prepayment plans such as Kaiser Permanente and Blue Cross and Blue Shield in the late 1930s and 1940s eventually countered the objections of the mainstream medical profession to contract practice, as growing numbers of Americans demanded affordable access to new medical technologies and therapies.[87] By the early 1950s, some colleges and universities had adopted or were considering adopting Blue Cross/Blue Shield programs. Others developed self-insurance plans or paid for student health services out of general tuition revenues. Unlike most other forms of health insurance, student health fees were nearly always compulsory, since they were founded on the concept that students lacked the knowledge or experience to purchase health care on their own.[88] As Ralph I. Canuteson, physician at the University of Kansas, observed in 1953, "We do not require a student to come to the University of Kansas if he doesn't want to." Those students choosing to attend the university, therefore, needed to adhere to policies regarding health fees, just as they were expected to follow parietal rules governing student behavior.[89]

The emphasis on prevention of disease and the educational functions of college and university health services eventually led the AMA to accept these centers as a legitimate alternative to state-sponsored forms of "socialized medicine" proposed during the Truman administration, which the AMA continued to oppose. The AMA's Bureau of Medical Economics conducted a follow-up study of university and college health services in 1949–50. Unlike the first survey in the 1930s, the authors insisted, "It is not our aim to pass judgment on any of the types of health services for college students, faculty members, and other employees and the methods for financing these surveys."[90] A decade later, the AMA emphatically endorsed the importance of college health services in "selling hygiene" to the American public. In 1959, the AMA House of Delegates accepted the recommendation of its Commission on Student Health Services that the "proper relationship between the medical profession and student health services should be one comprising study and participation; encouragement and understanding, and consultation and advice." In addition, the AMA recognized the "constructive efforts being made by educational institutions to provide medical service to students." Through its Department of Health Education, the AMA offered "all possible assistance" in ensuring good relations between local affiliates and student health services.[91]

Protection of the student body did not end with physical health. Indeed, efforts to improve the mental hygiene of college students evolved alongside these other public health movements and drew on them as models for disease prevention. As rates of physical illness declined, more attention focused on mental health issues such as depression, suicide, and alcohol abuse. Addressing these concerns would not only expand the mandate of college health services but also redefine the mission and purpose of institutions of higher education more generally.

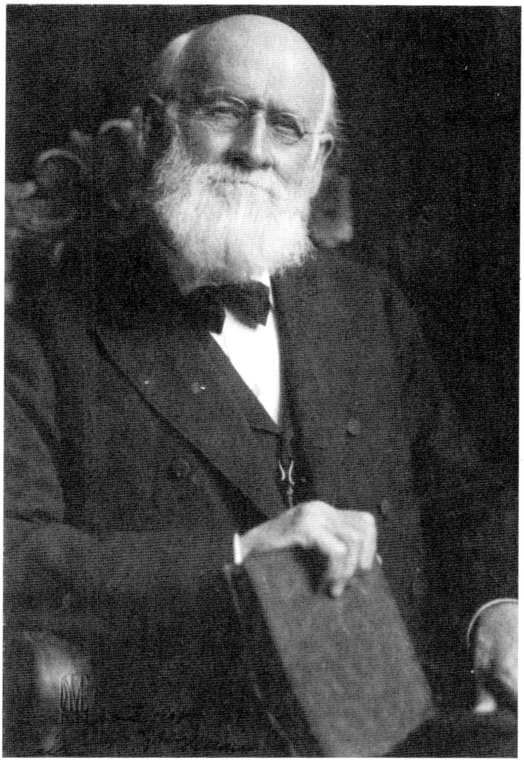

Dr. Edward C. Hitchcock Jr., professor of hygiene and physical education at Amherst College and one of the founding fathers of college health. In 1961, the centennial of Amherst College's hygiene program, the American College Health Association created the Edward C. Hitchcock award to commemorate his work and to honor association members who "have made outstanding contributions to advancing the health of all college students." *(Photograph courtesy of Amherst College Archives and Special Collections by permission of the Trustees of Amherst College.)*

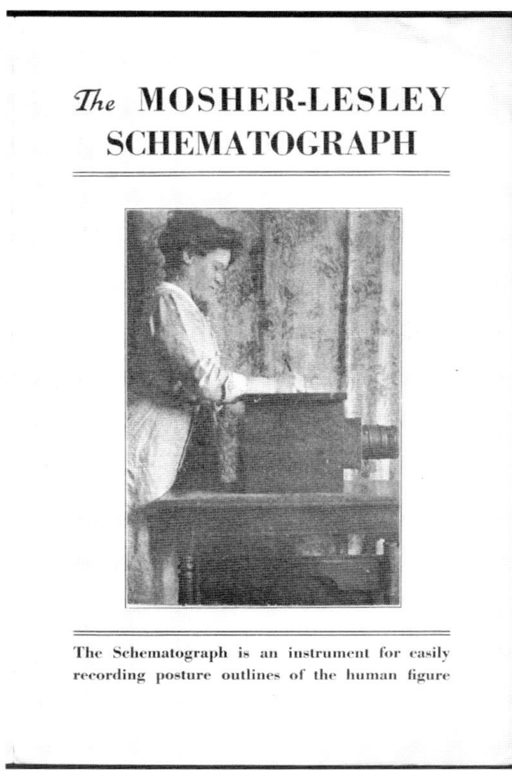

Physicians for women at female colleges and coeducational universities conducted anthropometric studies of their students to confirm that college life—and physical education in particular—improved rather than damaged women's bodies. This brochure touted the schematograph, an instrument designed by Dr. Clelia Duel Mosher at Stanford University to study posture and changes in bodily proportions. *(Photograph courtesy of Stanford University Archives.)*

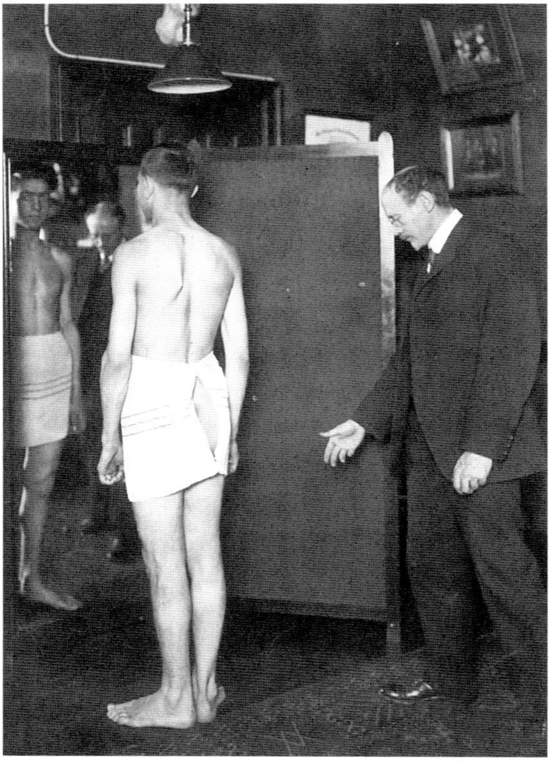

Male students also endured mandatory physical examinations and measurements of posture and muscular development. Here, Dr. R. Tait McKenzie examines a University of Pennsylvania student, ca. 1912. According to McKenzie, signs of impending race suicide were especially apparent in city dwellers like those who attended Penn. *(Photograph courtesy of Collections of the University of Pennsylvania Archives.)*

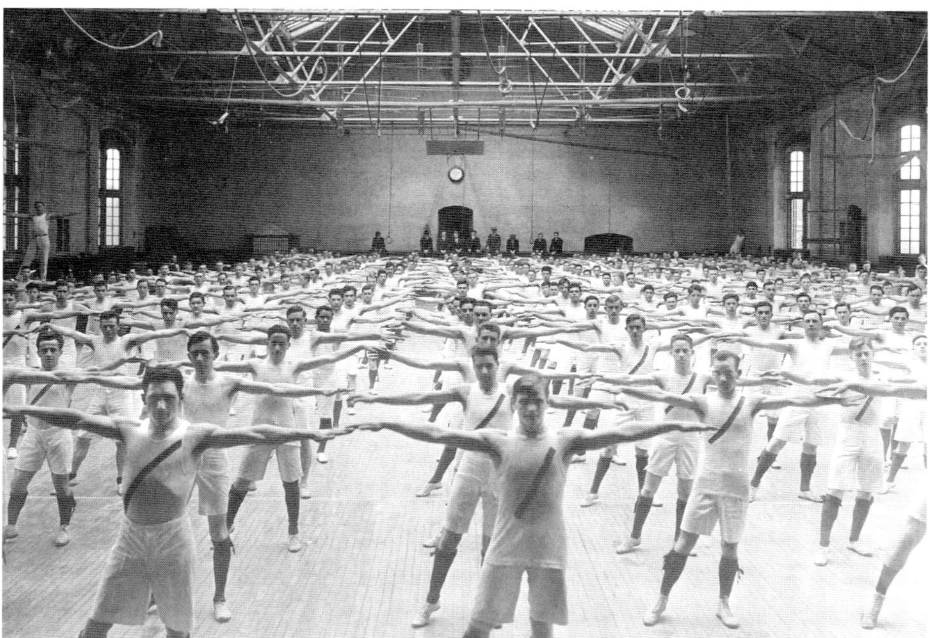

Many professional physical educators believed that mandatory exercise could compensate for the stress and strain of campus life and help build manly student bodies, as in this physical education class at the University of Pennsylvania, ca. 1905. *(Photograph courtesy of Collections of the University of Pennsylvania Archives.)*

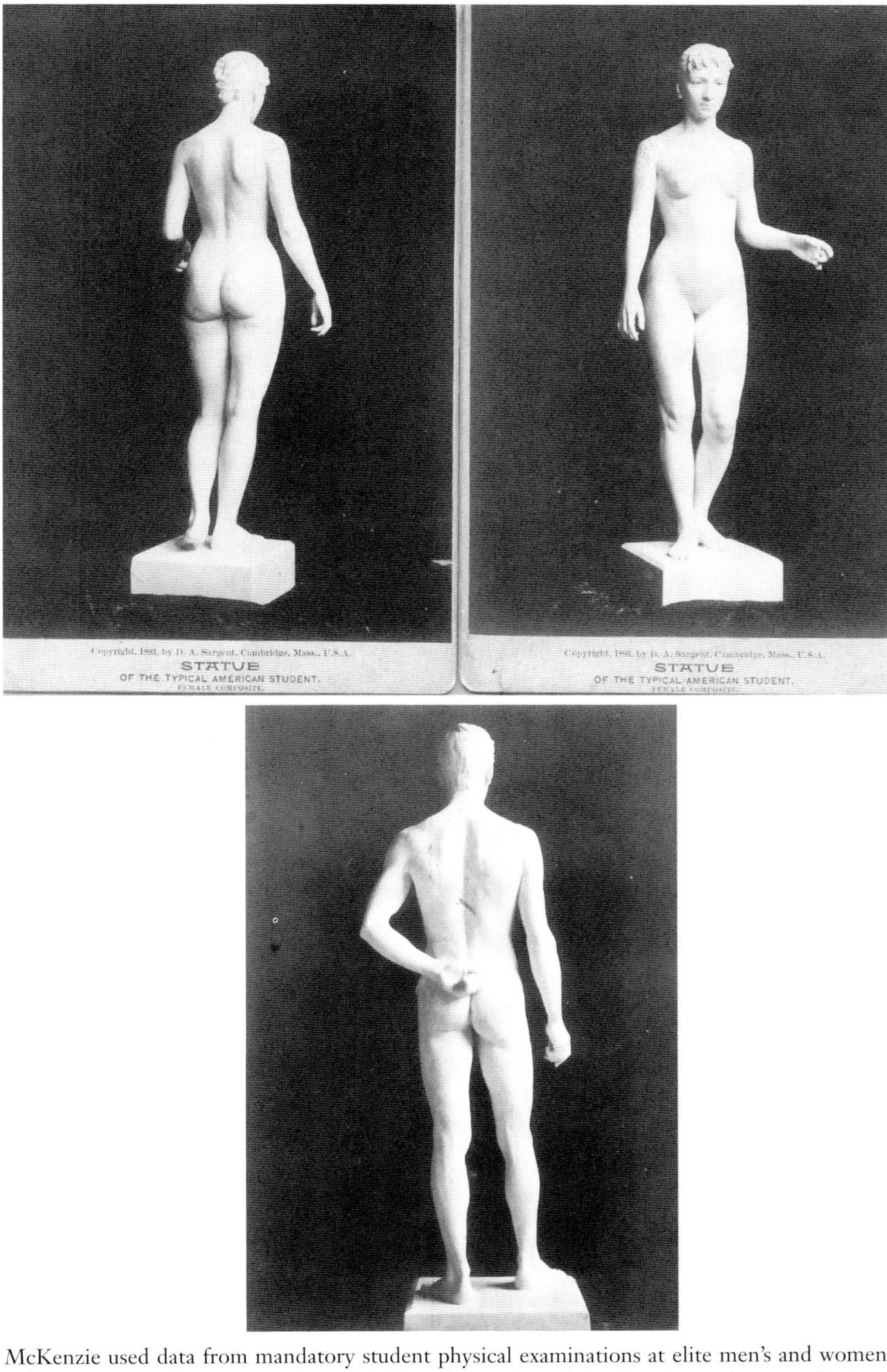

McKenzie used data from mandatory student physical examinations at elite men's and women's colleges to create these statues of "typical" American male and female students that were displayed at the 1893 Columbian World's Fair in Chicago. *(Photograph courtesy of Collections of the University of Pennsylvania Archives.)*

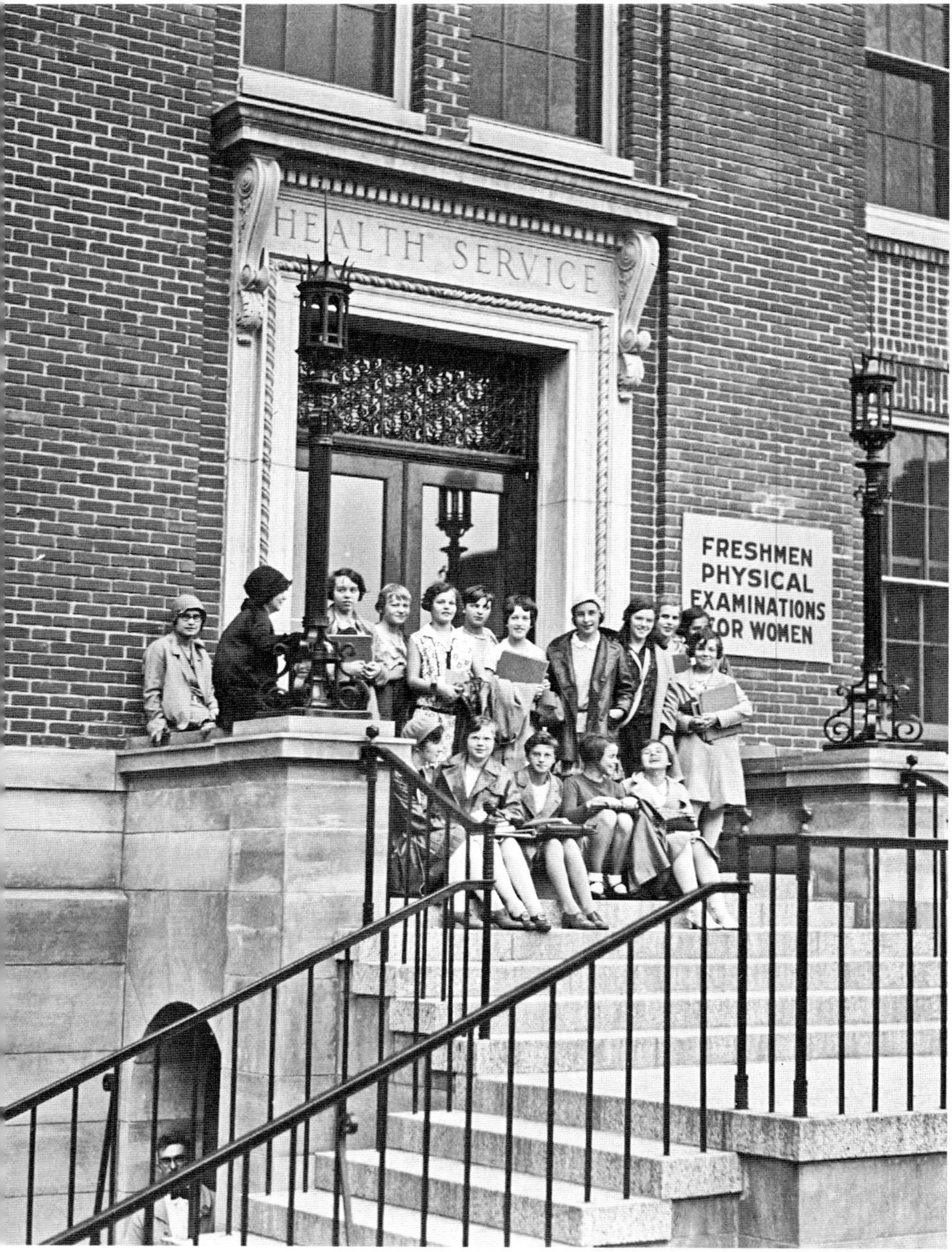

First-year women students at the University of Minnesota line up for mandatory physical examinations, ca. 1930s. During the Great Depression, many colleges and universities merged male and female health services in an attempt to cut costs. To justify their role in college health, women physicians continued to argue that female students had special needs and bodily differences that could only be addressed by female physicians. They also upheld female modesty to justify their work, claiming that it was inappropriate for male physicians to examine female students. *(Photograph courtesy of University of Minnesota Archives.)*

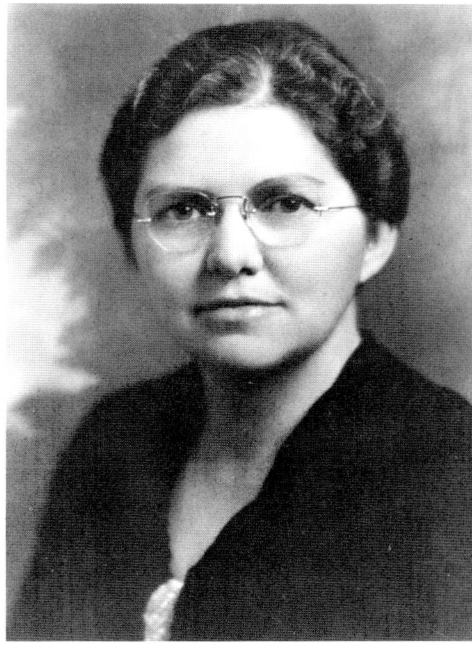

Ruth Evelyn Boynton, physician to women students at the University of Minnesota and charter member of the American Student Health Association. She served as executive secretary and was elected the organization's first female president in 1940. In 1967, the American College Health Association created the Boynton Award to honor members who have "provided distinguished service to the association." The Boynton Student Health Service at the University of Minnesota is named in her honor. *(Photograph courtesy of University of Minnesota Archives.)*

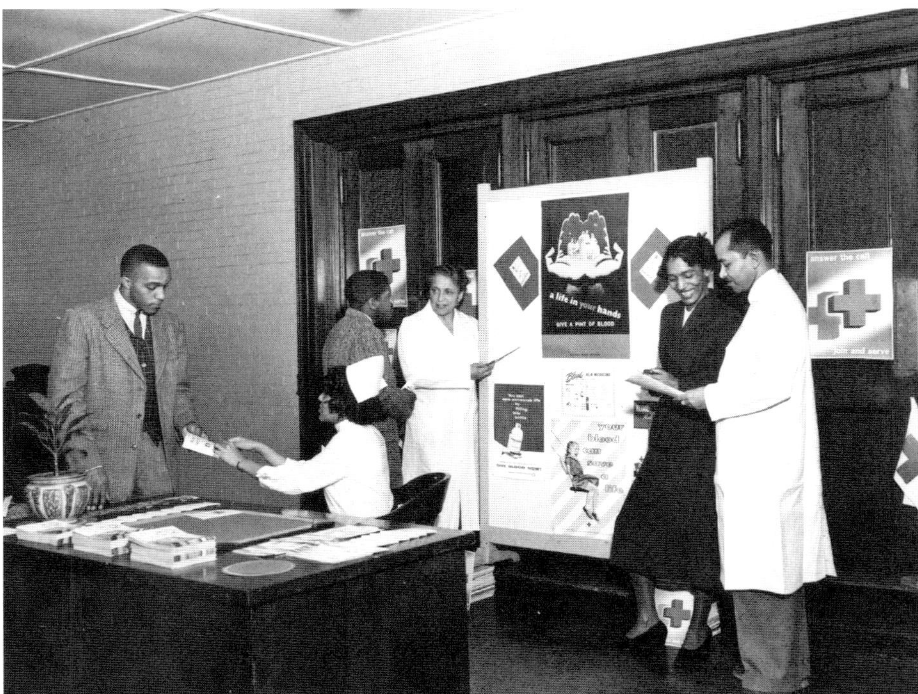
a life in your hands
answer the call
join and serve

The career of Dorothy Ferebee, standing, with pointer, shows the double burden that sexism and racism imposed on black women in medicine. Like other historically black institutions of higher education, Howard University provided more opportunities for women professionals than did other institutions. African American physicians emphasized the link between student health and racial uplift, using health care and hygiene instruction to improve the health conditions of African Americans as a whole. *(Photograph courtesy of Moorland-Spingarn Research Center, Howard University.)*

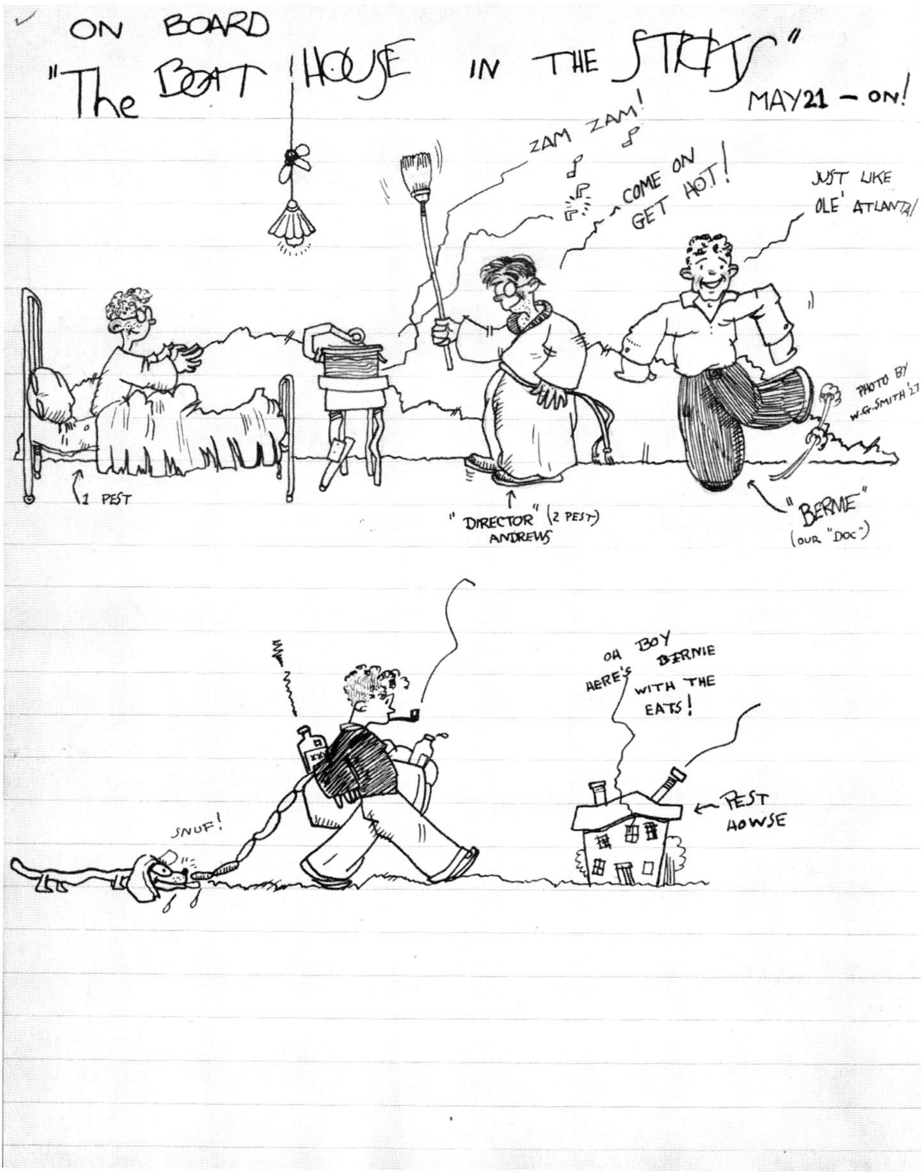

Dartmouth College students often used humor to describe their experiences at the notorious "Pest House," an isolation hospital on the outskirts of Hanover where those with contagious diseases were sent to avoid infecting the rest of the campus. *(Illustration from Isolation Hospital Logs, Rauner Special Collections, Dartmouth College Library. Courtesy of Dartmouth College Library.)*

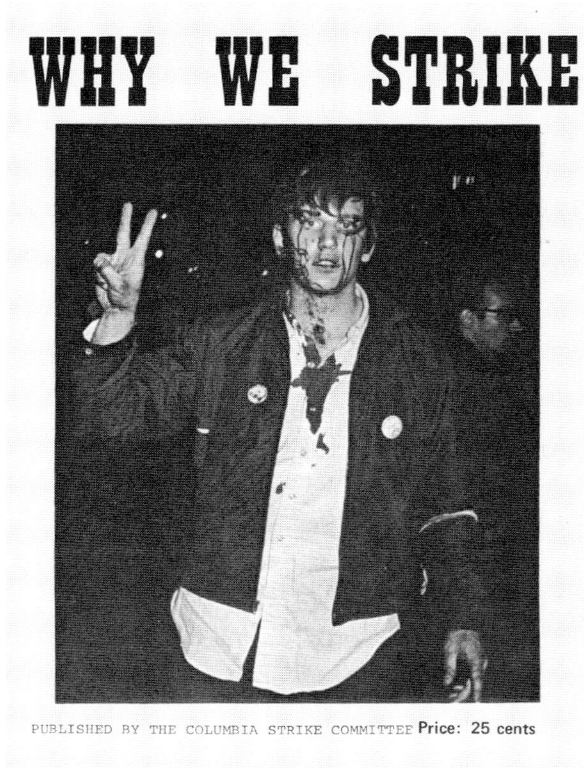

A Columbia University student injured by police during the 1968 strike protesting the campus presence of military and Central Intelligence Agency recruiters. During the 1960s, hundreds of young men and women put their bodies and lives in jeopardy in support of civil rights, disarmament, free speech, feminism, and an end to the war in Vietnam. Physicians on college campuses became accustomed to treating students injured during protests as well as to fielding increasing requests for advice on birth control, sexuality, and the use of illegal drugs. *(Photograph reproduced with permission of the University Archives, Columbia University in the City of New York.)*

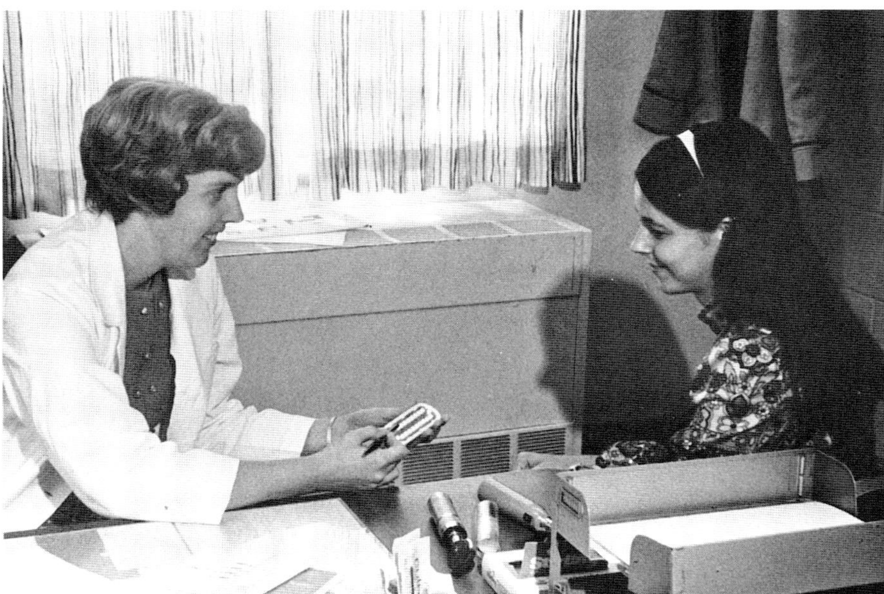

The University of Michigan was one of the earliest student health centers to prescribe contraceptives to women students regardless of marital status. *(Photograph [ca. 1968] from University Health Service Records, box 7, folder Photographs—Staff, Bentley Historical Library, University of Michigan. Courtesy of Bentley Historical Library, University of Michigan.)*

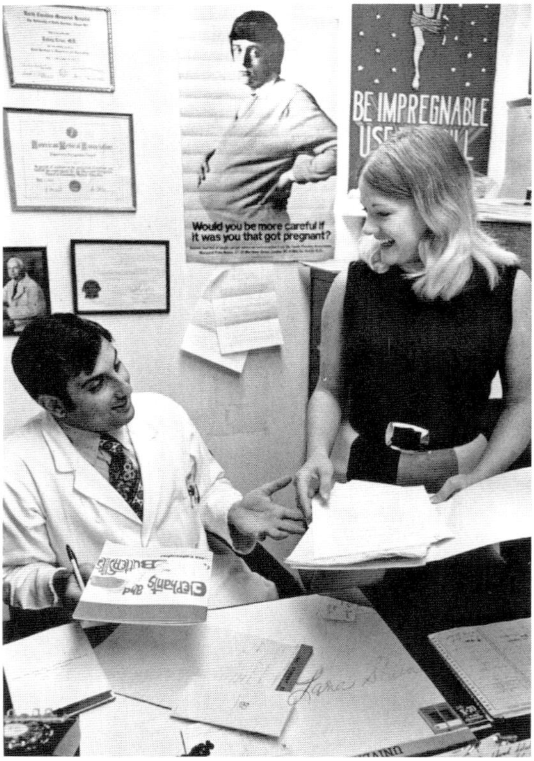
BE IMPREGNABLE
Would you be more careful if it was you that got pregnant?

University of North Carolina gynecologist Takey Crist and undergraduate Lana Starnes discuss the advice manual *Elephants and Butterflies*, ca. 1970. *(Photograph from Takey Crist Papers, courtesy of Rare Book, Manuscript, and Special Collections Library, Duke University.)*

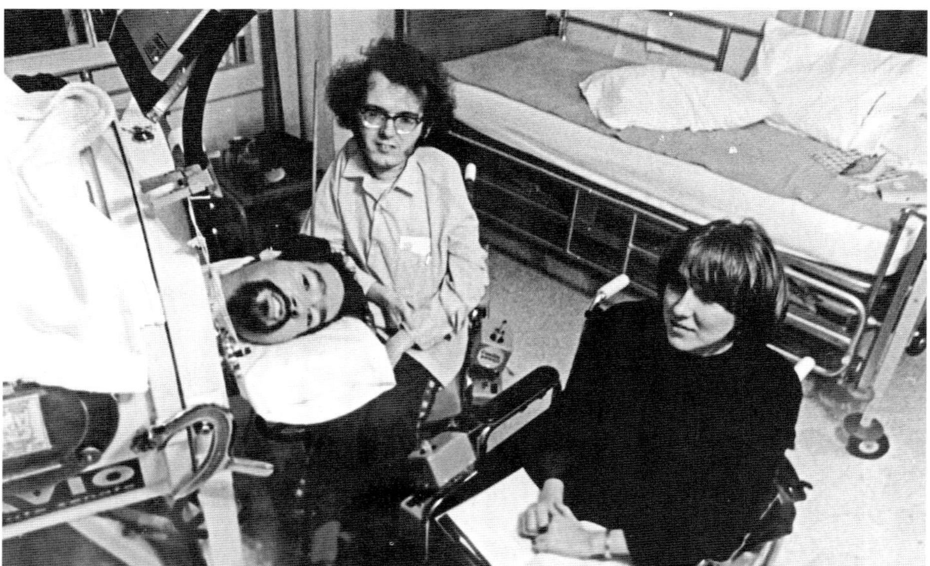

Ed Roberts and other residents of the Cowell Hospital Program for disabled students at the University of California, Berkeley, ca. 1968. Although the program allowed severely disabled students to attend the university, residents objected to the paternalism of staff members and formed a student rights organization, the Rolling Quads. Their activism led the university to create the Physically Disabled Students Program, the first "program for quads, run by quads." *(Photograph courtesy of Bancroft Library, University of California, Berkeley.)*

CHAPTER 6

Cultivating Mature Minds and Healthy Personalities

> A man's college days, collectively, are usually his happiest. Most of mine were not happy. Yet I look back upon them with great satisfaction, for I feel that I was fortunate enough to absorb some of that intangible but very real element known as the "Yale spirit." This has helped to keep Hope alive within me during my most discouraged moments, and now makes the accomplishment of my purpose seem easy and sure.
>
> —Clifford Whittingham Beers
> *A Mind That Found Itself* (1908)

Beers was not alone in his difficulties in handling the pressures of undergraduate life: many students in his time as well as today no doubt could identify with his descriptions of experiencing feelings of utter dread before examinations and class presentations. Beers's family physician, Dr. B. H. Cheney, had experience treating nervous ailments and prescribed sedatives so that Beers could finish his courses. Beers also had professors, who, when told of his condition, "invariably treated me with consideration." Yet this fact clearly burdened Beers, as he recalled that while his professors "never doubted the genuineness of my excuse, it was no easy matter to keep them convinced for almost two of the three years of my course."[1]

Other students at this time were less fortunate. Most faculty and administrators in the late nineteenth century, including those at Yale, would have dismissed Beers's symptoms as a sign that he was unfit for advanced study. Beers's affluence and family connections probably constituted crucial factors in his ability to win his instructors' cooperation. Not until 1910 did Dr. Stewart Paton, a psychiatrist and lecturer in neurobiology at Princeton University, start the first college mental hygiene service. Paton's work in neuropsychiatry led him to become interested in the emotional problems of undergraduates. After he invited all "troubled souls" to visit him with their problems, students reportedly flocked to see him by the dozens.[2]

Beers's memoir, likened to *Uncle Tom's Cabin* in its social impact, launched a nationwide mental hygiene movement aimed not only at improving the treatment of the mentally ill but also at early detection and prevention of mental and emotional disturbances. Isaac Ray, one of the founders of the American Psychiatric Association (APA), coined the term *mental hygiene* in 1893, defining it as the "art of preserving the mind against all incidents and influences calculated to deteriorate its qualities, impair its energies, or derange its movements." Preventive efforts included management of exercise, rest, food, clothing, and climate as well as learning to govern the "laws of breeding" and to "discipline of the intellect." According to Ray, all these factors and more "come within the province of mental hygiene."[3] Beers, along with like-minded progressives such as Paton and Adolph Meyer in psychiatry; G. Stanley Hall, William James, and James R. Angell in academic psychology; and Jane Addams and Julia Lathrop in social work, joined Beers in 1909 to form the National Committee for Mental Hygiene (NCMH). The formation of this organization was part of a larger "psychiatric renaissance" in the early twentieth century that sought to take psychiatry beyond the asylum walls and use the discipline to address problems in the home, the workplace, schools, and other social institutions. According to Meyer's concept of "maladjustment," mental disorders most often resulted from an individual's failure to fit into society.[4]

Beers was inspired by other progressive public health reforms of the early twentieth century, vowing to do for mental illness what had already been done for contagious diseases such as tuberculosis. Like the earlier social hygiene and antituberculosis movements, the NCMH aimed its preventive efforts at youth in schools and colleges in the belief that intervention was most effective during adolescence, when the personality was most malleable.[5] Professionals in college health likewise argued that institutions of higher educational were the most effective way to spread mental hygiene concepts throughout the nation.

Shell Shock and Student Stress

The work of military psychiatrists on shell shock and other psychoneuroses among soldiers during World War I provided a major theoretical underpinning for mental hygiene work in colleges and universities. NCMH medical director Thomas W. Salmon served as chief of the Division of Neuropsychiatry of the American Expeditionary Forces, where he became convinced that psychiatry was an important medical specialty "not only in times of war but also in times of peace."[6] During the war, Paton left Princeton to serve as a major in the medical corps on a commission to study shell shock. He also directed a unit that evaluated the psychological fitness of pilots for flight duty. After the war, Paton served as a lecturer in psychiatry at Columbia University, working closely with Salmon, Beers, Adolph Meyer, Frankwood Williams, and other members of the NCMH. This collaboration led to the 1917 creation of the national journal *Mental Hygiene*, which published numerous articles on the importance of mental hygiene in the college setting.[7]

Given the interest in shell shock in the armed forces, one of the first mental health services created after the war was at the U.S. Military Academy at West Point. The 1920 suicides of two cadets prompted the hiring of Dr. Harry N. Kerns to serve as the academy's psychiatrist and to conduct a study of the causes of common maladjustments among the cadets. Kerns found his experience with draftees during the war directly applicable to the training of regular officers at the academy. Kerns observed that the isolation, rigid discipline, and "almost total lack of opportunity for individual expression" at West Point contributed heavily to mental disorders among members of the cadet corps. Yet he also noted that the military academy could boast of "training in regular habits, an unparalleled physical education, excellent sanitary supervision, an *esprit de corps* second to none," and above all "training in honesty. Character in itself is not a safeguard against mental disease," Kerns admitted, "but if one is honest with one's fellows, one is more apt to be honest with oneself and to face one's problems squarely." Furthermore, faculty members' close surveillance of cadets meant that problems were detected early and reported promptly to the physician.[8]

According to Paton, the principles of mental hygiene learned during the war were directly applicable to students in civilian settings. "Peace no less than War produces 'shell shock,'" he wrote in *Education in War and Peace* (1920), a college textbook on mental hygiene. Although the war had prompted the military to "appreciate the necessity for protecting the soldier against shell-shock," Paton observed, very little had been done by colleges and universities "to protect the civilian in times of peace, by giving him the right kind of education to withstand the strain and stress of modern life."[9]

This situation would soon change, as a number of colleges and universities started mental hygiene programs. In 1920, Washburn College in Topeka, Kansas, hired Dr. Karl Menninger, another veteran of the Neuropsychiatry Division who had trained at Boston Psychopathic Hospital, to teach a course in mental hygiene and set up a counseling service for the students. The previous year, Menninger had established a group practice with his father, Charles, a general practitioner who realized that many of his patients suffered from nervous ailments despite no apparent physical illnesses. The Menningers would soon establish themselves as leaders in the "new psychiatry" that emphasized medical therapeutics over custodial care of the chronically mentally ill and focused on treating patients who suffered from less severe illnesses than those found in state hospitals. Karl Menninger was influenced by the work at Johns Hopkins University of Meyer, who stressed the importance of outreach to schools, churches, playgrounds, and other community agencies not only to prevent mental disorders but also to promote positive mental hygiene. Menninger believed that counseling college students was a "new phase of the application of dynamic and pragmatic psychiatry" similar to those established in public schools and child guidance clinics.[10]

In 1921, Dartmouth president Ernest Martin Hopkins consulted with Paton about creating a mental hygiene clinic at the college, believing "it is as legitimate a function of the College to stabilize minds and to make them healthful as it is to sharpen intellect." That year, Hopkins invited Arthur Hiler Ruggles (1903), superintendent of the Butler Psychiatric Hospital in Providence, Rhode Island, to serve as a psychiatric consultant to Dartmouth students. Ruggles had served in the Neuropsychiatry Division of the American Expeditionary Forces, a position that afforded him a "wonderful opportunity" to study large groups of men and their adjustments to various situations, work that continued once these men were discharged. "To work on such a problem at Dartmouth—a place which has an unusual hold on me both through my own associations and that of my forbears," Ruggles wrote to Hopkins, "seems almost like the fulfillment of a long standing but unexpressed ambition."[11]

Other elite colleges soon followed Dartmouth's example. Vassar College was the first women's college to recognize the need for mental hygiene, which President Henry N. MacCracken saw as a natural extension of the college's historic interest in controlling the campus environment to promote hygiene. In 1923, MacCracken asked neurologist Austen Fox Riggs, founder of a successful psychiatric hospital in Stockbridge, Massachusetts, and a national expert on shell shock, to serve as a mental hygiene consultant. Riggs reported that he and his associate, William B. Terhune, had the full support of faculty and key administrators, including MacCracken, Dean C. Mildred Thompson, and college physician Elizabeth Burr Thelberg. Riggs and Terhune also counted members of the student government among their strongest supporters. The college soon realized it needed a full-time resident psychiatrist to handle emergencies as well as regular treatment. Since there was a shortage of trained psychiatrists at this time and competition for them was fierce, Thelberg allowed her associate physician, Dr. Anaple Christie, to take a leave of absence to pursue psychiatric training. The college also hired Dr. Smiley Blanton, a psychiatrist and child guidance expert from Minnesota, to teach courses in mental hygiene within the college's euthenics division.[12] Not to be outdone, other elite women's colleges such as Smith, Wellesley, Pembroke, Bryn Mawr, and Radcliffe soon imitated Vassar's program.[13]

Yale started a mental hygiene clinic in 1925 as part of a larger effort to establish a department of psychiatry in the medical school. Influenced by the Meyer's work, medical school dean Milton C. Winternitz saw a need for a new type of medical practice that paid as much attention to an individual's personality as to his organs. Winternitz also wanted medicine to become more oriented toward prevention and the community, urging physicians to view the patient as a whole rather than a collection of individual parts. Winternitz persuaded Ruggles to leave Dartmouth in 1925 and become Yale's first professor of psychiatry and mental hygiene consultant to the students. The following year, Winternitz applied for a grant from the Commonwealth Fund, a leading nonprofit agency that financed a variety of training programs and demonstration projects in mental hygiene throughout the early twentieth century. The fund's director, Barry C. Smith, believed that the Yale program held the promise of answering important, unsolved questions about the best way to establish mental hygiene for college students and thereby aid other colleges and universities "in the intelligent establishment of mental hygiene services." The fund granted Yale fifty thousand dollars per year for five years, allowing the department to hire Kerns and Paton along with two other psychiatrists, Clement Fry and Lloyd Thompson, as well as several social workers.[14]

In the late 1920s, the University of Pennsylvania started a college personnel service as an extension of the Psychological Clinic, a child guidance center started by psychology professor Lightner Witmer in 1896. Like other child guidance clinics, the one at Pennsylvania had started as an adjunct to the juvenile court system and as such was initially interested in the causes of juvenile delinquency. By the early 1920s, the clinic was attracting a growing number of middle- and upper-class parents from the Philadelphia area who sought help dealing with their children's "problem" behavior. The college service was a natural extension of the clinic's interest in reaching a more socioeconomically and ethnically diverse clientele. Consequently, many of the clients at this clinic were University of Pennsylvania students.[15] Within a few years, these private institutions were joined by large state universities such as the Universities of Michigan, Minnesota, California, Vermont, and Wyoming. By the end of the decade, at least twenty private and public colleges and universities had added mental hygiene to their health services on at least a part-time basis.[16]

The College Is Not a Sanitarium

Establishing mental hygiene on the college level was not smooth, however. Because of its historical roots in the asylum, psychiatry had a low professional status compared to other branches of medicine at this time. Mental illnesses—even minor ones—still carried an overwhelming social stigma. The eugenics movement reinforced preexisting notions that psychiatric patients were physically and mentally defective.[17] Faculty members were skeptical of mental hygienists, believing them to be coddling students who could not meet academic standards. A survey of college mental hygienists conducted in 1928 found the faculty the "greatest hindrance to the success of the college mental hygiene program."[18]

Even colleges with well-established mental hygiene services initially hesitated to let the public know about their work until the field gained more scientific and popular legitimacy. At Dartmouth, President Hopkins told the associate editor of the social work journal the *Survey* in 1924 that he was not certain whether it was wise to give much publicity to the school's mental hygiene program until more data demonstrated its effectiveness. More importantly, he had the challenge of "disabusing the minds of those who are inclined to think of us as running a sanitorium [*sic*]." In fact, Hopkins reported, he was "appalled" when approached by a father who wanted to send his "mentally defective" son to Dartmouth. "I need not elaborate on the feelings of a Dartmouth official at the thought of the work developing along this line and having this effect upon the minds of parents," Hopkins wrote.[19]

This popular conflation of mental illness and mental "defectiveness" was all too common, even as the mental hygiene movement attempted to stress that most emotional problems were treatable, especially if caught early. The development of the Stanford-Binet Intelligence Quotient (IQ) test and its widespread use to screen World War I recruits revealed that the average intelligence of the American population was shockingly low, particularly among recent immigrants, the poor, and African Americans. Although these findings were controversial at the time, many members of the general public feared that the country was being overrun by "idiots" and "morons." Psychologists and psychiatrists used "mental defects" to explain the growing incidence of crime, illegitimacy, juvenile delinquency, and other social ills in early-twentieth-century American society. In some quarters, these claims fueled existing social and racial prejudices, seeming to provide a scientific basis for immigration restriction, sterilization, and other extreme measures aimed at ridding the country of the alleged menace posed by the "feebleminded."[20]

Admissions directors at elite colleges hoped these new psychometric tests could be used to weed out "undesirable" social groups, especially Jews. Much to their dismay, however, admissions officers found that Jewish students tended, on average, to excel at admissions tests and other measures of intellectual ability.[21] Furthermore, intelligence tests alone did not predict success in college. During the 1920s and 1930s, physicians in college health services called attention to a disturbing trend: increasing numbers of apparently bright students were dropping out because of emotional difficulties. A previous generation would have dismissed these "academic casualties" as representatives of an inferior grade of student, but by the 1920s, many of those involved in student health services and student personnel work began to challenge that idea. Many mental hygienists believed that the most severe cognitive impairments and mental illnesses had a hereditary basis but tried to counter this pessimism by suggesting that most mental problems—particularly those in young people—resulted from environmental factors. Drawing on Sigmund Freud's psychodynamic theories, mental hygiene experts argued that the "troublesome" behavior of children and youth could be attributed to "maladjustments" between the individual and his or her environment. Believing childhood was the "period *par excellence* for prophylaxis," mental hygiene experts called for early intervention in the home, the school, and the community.[22]

Taking this concept a step further, mental hygiene experts in colleges and universities argued that young adulthood was the last opportunity to detect and prevent mental illnesses. According to Menninger, counseling of college students "may be viewed as the facilitation of personality development at a critical point, comparable to a bad turn on a race track." Faculty and deans could help students negotiate this "critical curve in character development" by "watching for impending spills" and "ominous indications in the driver's technique or equipment." Menninger advocated employing skilled college-level counselors to demonstrate to faculty and administrators the "possibility of averting some of the spills and crashes" and to correct "unpropitious trends and errors in adaptations to the track."[23] Because of the dramatic expansion in college attendance following the war, mental hygienists at both private and public institutions found themselves trying to explain the behavior of an increasingly diverse college population. Interest in "better breeding" among college students ensured that concerns about sexuality and gender identity played a prominent role in mental hygienists' work with this age group.

Mental Hygiene and the "Homosexual Menace"

By the 1920s, concerns about heterosexual relationships were outweighed by fears about a different sort of "sexual danger" facing undergraduates—homosexuality. As early as 1903, Hall had warned in his classic *Adolescence* about the psychological dangers of "smashing," or passionate, romantic friendships between girls and young women that were common at female schools and colleges during the nineteenth and early twentieth centuries.[24] Developmental psychologists in the 1910s and 1920s alleged that single-sex environments posed the same dangers for young men. These experts acknowledged that a temporary homosexual phase in childhood and adolescence was common and even protected boys and girls from premature sexual experimentation but agreed that persistence of homosexual tendencies into late adolescence and early adulthood was pathological. Williams, for example, warned that heterosexuality "does not just happen; it is a development and growth that is nourished and contained by what it feeds upon."[25]

Kerns observed that as a result of West Point's "reputation for making men," the academy attracted "a large group of youngsters (larger, perhaps, than obtains at any civilian school) who have been made to feel that they fall short of this manly standard." While "most of this group really makes excellent compensations," Kerns observed, "if for any reason the compensation breaks, there is serious trouble ahead." Moreover, the "monastic environment of West Point" was "highly conducive to frank sex problems" since there was "practically no opportunity for normal sex expression at West Point, and furlough comes but once in four years." Despite this risk, Kerns had "never met a conscious homosexual problem among the cadets" because "a great many have found excellent sublimations for unconscious homosexual tendencies" through athletics and other physical activities. It was usually the "partially sublimated types" who made up a "considerable of the depressions and psychoneuroses." Kerns added that the sex problem about which he was most frequently consulted was masturbation, with many students suffering from "misinformation and fear" about the allegedly "evil" consequences of autoeroticism. In these cases, he wrote, "treatment is simply a matter of removing the element of fear by a candid statement of truth." Kerns claimed to have prevented at least three suicides by reassuring cadets that masturbation was a safe and natural outlet for normal adolescent sexual feelings.[26]

Concerns about homosexuality were also prevalent at elite male colleges, which by the 1920s were facing growing public allegations that they were havens for "pansies" and "queers." The suicides of two homosexual students at Harvard in 1920 revealed a gay male subculture linking Harvard undergraduates with other homosexuals in Cambridge and Boston. Whereas previous college administrators had been more concerned about keeping prostitutes out of the Harvard dormitories and the Yard, President A. Lawrence Lowell and Dean Chester N. Greenough used the 1920 suicides as an excuse to rid the campus once and for all of its "nest of perverts." Lowell appointed a "secret court," which included hygiene professor and health service director Roger I. Lee, to investigate the extent to which homosexuality had permeated undergraduate life.[27] This "homosexual panic" extended to other members of the "big three"—Yale and Princeton—who also worried they were attracting too many "sissies." To remedy this problem, these institutions reaffirmed their commitment to physical examinations of entering students and mandatory physical education for all undergraduates. They also began using measures other than intelligence as admissions standards. In addition to evaluating academic credentials, admissions officials enlisted the help of health service staff to assess the "personality" and "character" of applicants. Administrators were especially interested in finding students who were "manly" and sufficiently "sound of mind, body, and spirit" to serve as future leaders.[28]

This growing emphasis on "manliness" and "emotional stability" intersected with another perceived "menace" to elite male colleges—Jewish applicants. Some mental health experts claimed that Jewish students' allegedly superior intellectual abilities actually made them more prone to mental disturbances and sexual perversions. Dr. Charles W. Burr, chair of mental diseases at the University of Pennsylvania Hospital and a pioneer in the study of schizophrenia, wrote in *Hygeia* in 1928 that Jews were often precocious in childhood but fell behind children of the "Nordic" race by the time they reached adolescence and adulthood. "The precocious boy," Burr warned, "often becomes an eccentric and not infrequently breaks during adolescence." Burr added that he had noticed in his rounds of mental hospitals an "astonishing number of men with long tapering fingers, effeminate in type," although there was no "corresponding anatomic abnormality in mentally ill girls."[29]

These anti-Semitic stereotypes were reinforced by the infamous "trial of the century" involving Nathan Leopold Jr. and Richard Loeb, two young University of Chicago students from wealthy German-Jewish families who in 1924 kidnapped and murdered Loeb's fourteen-year-old second cousin, Bobby Franks. Rather than plead not guilty by reason of insanity, the young men's defense team, led by Clarence Darrow, called in the nation's child mental hygiene experts to gain a lighter sentence for his clients based on "mitigating circumstances." The trial reinforced theories that explicitly linked Jewishness, precocious intellectual ability, homosexuality, and mental instability. Yet the defense testimony also drove home the notion that even highly intelligent, economically privileged youths of "good family heritage" could become mentally unstable as a result of warped family situations and faulty child-rearing practices. Noted child guidance expert William Healy testified that little difference existed between the defendants and the many "very innocent children of fine people" he saw in his practice, children who got into all sorts of mischief short of murder yet still grew up in "very nice ways." According to Healy, Leopold and Loeb's "depraved" acts simply represented an extreme version of the "everyday problems of the everyday child."[30]

At women's colleges, mental hygienists faced the dilemma of discouraging homosexual relationships while reinforcing sexual propriety. Vassar's Dean Thompson wrote of the problems caused by the "week-end habit" of Vassar students traveling to social events at men's colleges (with chaperones, of course). "For the week-end habitués come the exhaustion and shattering drabness of the Monday morning after, with mental and physical fag quite inadequate to the accumulations of reading and topics that somehow have not got themselves done." Equally worrisome was the girl "who is left behind," who "hasn't boy friends to come over for solace" and for whom there was nothing but "envy and desolation and a sense of failure." In either event, Thompson observed, "the right-and-wrong categories of conventional morality do not go to the root of the trouble and do not help the young person get insight into her emotional disturbance." Unless the college took a straightforward and honest approach toward sexual questions, "there may be only concealment, not removal of the conflict and consequent distress."[31]

At Smith College, Dr. Florence Meredith observed that "unnatural" relationships between students were rare. Yet she also warned that certain homosexual tendencies in the faculty or staff could have a damaging effect on students. "The attitude of abhorrence of youthful interest in mating is quite as unsatisfactory in a college as an overtly homosexual attitude," she wrote. Such "unresolved" homosexual tendencies are "responsible for many of the unnecessarily strict regulations." Although some rules were needed to prevent scandalous behavior, she admitted, it was important that they did not "become too restrictive and do not too closely confine the student who is justifiably seeking to find scope for all her normal interests and powers."[32]

For guidance on how to protect the morals of young women while preventing homosexuality, mental hygienists looked to new ideas about the psychology of girls and women promoted by feminist-oriented social scientists such as Jessie Taft, Margaret Mead, Leta Hollingworth, Phyllis Blanchard, and Helen Thompson Woolley as well as by birth control advocates such as Margaret Sanger and Mary Ware Dennett. These theories rejected nineteenth-century views about female sexual purity, making heterosexual longings a normal part of female sexual development, albeit one fraught with peril. Dennett even argued that old-fashioned prudery and shame regarding sexual matters caused more harm than good. By presenting sex as vulgar and immoral, Dennett argued, parents and educators caused young women to rebel by snatching "at some of the outward aspects of freedom" while ignorant of the "fine flowering and full fruitage of balanced sexual living." Dennett's proposed solution was for sex educators to help girls and women acknowledge their sexual desires but enable them to have the confidence to resist or at least limit male sexual advances.[33] Although Dennett's ideas remained controversial among some educators, others incorporated her pamphlet, *The Sex Side of Life*, into courses in hygiene, physical education, home economics, biology, marriage and family, and child study. Professors at Connecticut's New Britain Normal School included the publication in a bibliography of materials recommended for future teachers of home economics in public schools. The student counselor for the Student Christian Association at the University of Michigan called the pamphlet the "best presentation for adolescent youth that I have ever come across." Students too were eager to read Dennett's work. Grinnell College education professor Milton Wittler noted that following a student presentation in his class, the book "has begun passing from hand to hand with the promise of becoming speedily dog-eared from much use."[34]

Yet limits existed to what experts considered normal sexual curiosity and experimentation. Single-sex institutions handled the problem of homosexuality by inviting undergraduates from select men's colleges to campus for carefully supervised social events and allowing female students the privilege of attending similarly chaperoned activities at male institutions. Increased automobile ownership among wealthy college students facilitated the practice of men and women visiting each other's campuses. However, student handbooks spelled out increasingly elaborate parietal rules regarding interaction between men and women. In general, campuses regulated student conduct by restricting the movement of women students and imposing various fines and penalties for violating rules about male visitors, chaperones, and curfews and other measures aimed at upholding reputable social standards. Since these rules did not prohibit sex per se but merely made it more difficult for men and women to get together, college authorities also relied on women students to set limits on what was appropriate. Although these peer group standards condoned kissing and the new practice of "petting," they still retained a sexual double standard in which "nice" girls waited until they were married or at least engaged before they "went all the way."[35]

Mental hygienists' concerns about normal sexual development fit well with efforts to establish sex education programs on college campuses. According to social hygienist Max Exner, parietal rules and other "special protective measures" were by themselves "only palliative." Equally if not more important were "internal safeguards of personality and character." Although ideally such "sex-character training lies in the home because of the formative character of the early years," Exner argued, "more progress than anywhere else has been made in the universities and colleges." Exner believed this was the best course of action because through the "educators and leaders of public opinion in the making, which we have in the colleges, the home situation will come to be influenced more rapidly than if the attention had been directed exclusively to the present generation of parents." For this reason, Exner called on institutions of higher education to take more responsibility for "preparing students for the most important responsibilities of life, namely marriage, parenthood, and home-making." Exner proposed that all colleges and universities offer courses for juniors and seniors presenting the "more intimate matters of sex in marriage such as must be understood as a basis of successful adjustment and happiness in married life."[36] Thus, sex education programs, in the form of family life education, sought not only to control the spread of venereal disease but also to eradicate the "homosexual menace" on campus.

Manpower and Mindpower

Experiences with psychiatric problems in the military during World War II heightened interest in the mental hygiene of young people. Shortly after the United States entered the war, Fry published *Mental Health in the College*, an analysis of problems presented to the Yale Mental Hygiene Division since the service started in 1925. Fry stressed that "all but a few of the patients treated by a college mental hygiene department are so-called 'normal' boys" and that the "problems which disturb them emotionally and physically arise in the normal process of their growth and in their adaptation to the special environment of a college or university." Fry argued that colleges should realize that for many students, "carefree college days are a myth" and should accept "responsibility for the emotional health" of students. These obligations "should go further than helping the more obvious misfits to find a secure place in the life of the college group," Fry argued. Instead, a college "should recognize the universality among its students of problems associated with growth and transition."[37]

To study this problem, Fry and his associates contracted with the National Research Council's Office of Scientific Research and Development to examine the military experience of 1,198 former mental hygiene patients at Yale and 819 former patients of the Harvard clinic. The results of the study confirmed the usefulness of mental hygiene programs on the college level. Fry found that the majority of former patients successfully adjusted to military life and that their rate of discharge was no greater than those who had not experienced emotional problems while in college. On the contrary, Fry observed, those with previous experience with psychiatry had more insight into their personalities and showed more resilience under stress than did other recruits. Fry found that existing methods of screening were not very effective in preventing psychiatric casualties. Many students whom evaluators predicted would succumb to combat stress actually adapted quite well; conversely, apparently "normal" recruits suffered mental breakdowns.[38]

In 1945, Fry argued that his wartime studies indicated that the college age was a distinct branch of psychiatry, requiring and deserving "special study" so that "young people may realize their full potentialities through education, and become capable of making successful and productive adjustments in society." He noted that "the college environment is an ideal setting for observation and study" of the problems of youth, since it could "be thoroughly documented; some areas can even be manipulated for special purposes." Although college students represented a "privileged and restricted group," Fry argued, they made up the majority of officer candidates. Furthermore, the G.I. Bill was causing "a considerable shift in the social makeup of the college community," even at elite institutions such as Yale. All of these factors, Fry concluded, pointed to the usefulness of "Yale materials as particular instances representing universal problems of youth in our culture."[39]

Psychiatrists who served in the military shared Fry's observations. More than 2.5 million men and women were rejected or discharged from military service for emotional problems. Most troubling was the high incidence of psychiatric problems that occurred in men who had shown no previous signs of mental disturbance. According to Brigadier General William C. Menninger, Karl's younger brother and chief of the U.S. Army's Neuropsychiatric Division, "those of us most intimately connected with the examination and treatment of these men and women were greatly harassed and distressed. We had neither the manpower nor the knowledge to do the job that should have been done. Understandably, we looked in every possible direction for help." He and other military psychiatrists first appealed to the APA for guidance, appearing before the APA Council to express their concerns. "Although the members of the Council were concerned and sympathetic," Menninger recalled, the APA "had neither the organizational structure nor the manpower to be helpful to us."[40] More importantly, the organization was oriented primarily around hospital psychiatry and somatic treatments and showed little interest in mental hygiene or dynamic psychiatry. Menninger and his supporters therefore had to look for a new avenue for their efforts to address the mental hygiene issues of postwar students.

The Group for the Advancement of Psychiatry Committee on the College Student

In 1946, William Menninger led a group of thirteen psychoanalytically trained psychiatrists and founded the Group for the Advancement of Psychiatry (GAP), which tried to reorient the profession toward community-based models of treatment and social activism. GAP spoke out on major social issues of the day, publishing a number of position papers condemning maltreatment of the mentally ill, shock treatment, psychosurgery, and segregation, which they believed was a major factor in emotional problems found among African Americans. The group also believed that a multidisciplinary approach, incorporating the work of clinical psychiatrists, social workers, and interested physicians from other specialties, was the best way to meet the "Herculean tasks of reconstruction and expansion" of mental health services on both the military and civilian fronts following the war. Within a month of its founding, GAP received a seventeen thousand dollar grant from the Commonwealth Fund to defray expenses and encourage the organization to expand its scope as far as possible. The organization also received critical support from the Rockefeller Foundation, with Dr. Alan Gregg, director of the foundation's Division of Medical Sciences, serving as an honorary GAP member. Gregg's participation in and support of GAP represented his firm commitment to both psychiatry and public health as well as his desire to expand the place of psychiatry in the medical curriculum. Like the prewar mental hygiene movement, members of GAP believed prevention and public awareness were the best ways to combat the problem of mental illness. They therefore targeted much of their efforts at improving child and adolescent mental hygiene in schools and colleges.[41]

The 1947 report issued by President Truman's Commission on Higher Education lent further support to the idea of improving mental hygiene in colleges and universities. The report argued that "for a satisfying and successful life[,] a person must also be emotionally stable and mature, able to endure the conflicts and tensions, the compromises and defeats, that life is most certain to bring." Therefore, colleges and universities not only should train the intellect but also "should make growth in emotional and social adjustment one of its major aims." The report concluded that to do so, students should receive adequate instruction in the sciences of human behavior as well as guidance and practice on how to apply this knowledge in everyday life.[42]

By the early 1950s, college presidents were also expressing growing interest in mental hygiene. In 1953, President J. L. Morrill of the University of Minnesota sent a survey to 200 other presidents of colleges or universities around the country asking for their most pressing health issues on their campuses. More than half of the 116 respondents said that emotional problems were the most prevalent health issues on their campuses. Poor health habits involving diet, sleep, and rest—all of which contributed to or exacerbated mental health problems—constituted the second-largest category of concern. Yet according to ACHA president and Harvard University health service director Dana Farnsworth, only slightly more than 100 of the country's 1,887 colleges and universities offered mental health services.[43]

Farnsworth played a leading role in expanding mental hygiene on college campuses. A 1933 graduate of Harvard Medical School, Farnsworth began his career as assistant director of health services at Williams College, where he established close professional contacts with psychiatrists at both Yale and Vassar and made mental hygiene a central part of the health program. During the war, Farnsworth served as chief of psychiatry aboard the USS *Solace* and at the U.S. Naval Hospital in Bethesda, Maryland, and contributed data on Williams College students serving in the military to Fry's study for the National Research Council.[44] After the war, Farnsworth accepted a position as a psychiatrist in the health service at the Massachusetts Institute of Technology and served on the GAP Committee on Academic Education, organized by William Menninger to study the state of college mental hygiene and to serve as a "nucleus in organized psychiatry" for those involved in college mental hygiene work.[45]

The first result of the committee's efforts was a report, *The Role of Psychiatrists in Colleges and Universities*, that reiterated the need to expand mental hygiene programs in institutions of higher education. Despite the general increase in public interest in psychiatry over the previous thirty years, the report observed, "many educators are either unaware of psychiatry or not certain what role the psychiatrist may play on the college campus." Although college students represented a small percentage of American youth, "college graduates form a high percentage of the leaders of any community, and the more maturity they display in their leadership the better it is for the community." Furthermore, the report asserted, the "emotional problems of late adolescence can be reached more effectively in a relatively brief period—in other words, the late adolescent can often make very constructive use of treatment." Those who dropped out because of emotional difficulties represented a "real loss to society in terms of educated service and citizenry." More importantly, students with "emotional handicaps" who did not drop out carried these problems into their later family and community lives, further contributing to the incidence of mental illness in the adult population and increasing the number of children and adolescents raised by "maladjusted" parents. The report concluded with a call for colleges and universities to "explicitly broaden their educational concepts to include the attainment of emotional maturity in addition to the normal goal of intellectual development." To do so, psychiatrists must head a "coordinated team effort" consisting of psychologists, sociologists, psychiatric social workers, and other "counselors of students" including deans and faculty. "The time has come when no institution of higher learning can perform its optimum service without taking psychiatric principles into consideration," the report declared.[46]

Several years later, the committee, now renamed the Committee on the College Student, issued a follow-up report offering advice to faculty and administrators on the best ways to encourage students' personality development. "The fostering of mature personalities can be regarded as the main promise of modern psychiatry," they committee members wrote. Yet the environment of modern higher education complicated the process of late adolescent/young adult maturation. "Our society, with its pattern of prolonged education, together with the occasional overprotectiveness of parents, tends to foster dependency," the report observed. "This clashes with the growing urge toward independent, self-directing activity," which mental health experts believed was the major sign of adult maturity. "This conflict," the group warned, "may be manifested in rebellious behavior," including "defiance toward parents or college authorities" as manifested in such reckless acts as excessive drinking, drag racing, vandalism, riots, and sexual escapades.[47] College authorities did not need to be reminded of troublesome antics of postwar undergraduates, problems that only became more prevalent as the college population expanded dramatically following the war. The G.I. Bill and a flourishing postwar economy drew a more ethnically and socioeconomically diverse student population to the nation's campuses than ever before, with many first-generation students using higher education as a ticket to the middle class. Officials in higher education, especially those in public institutions, found themselves dealing with a larger and more heterogeneous population. Male students, who already enjoyed considerably more freedoms than women, became more difficult to control after the war. Returning veterans, who were older and had more worldly experience than the average male college student of earlier decades, were especially reluctant to submit to supervision of their activities outside the classroom. Psychological literature warned of the dangers of robbing men of the "deep and perfectly normal masculine drives" permitted during the war. Deans and presidents were all too happy to turn over the responsibility of student disciplinary issues to college mental hygienists, believing that their experience "in evaluating and managing large groups of young people" was directly relevant to the college environment. At the same time, many campus authorities drew on new theories about late adolescent development, proposing that the purpose of college education was to develop "mature" and "responsible" citizens capable of making their own decisions.[48] This new approach to managing campus life was especially apparent in attempts to control undergraduate alcohol use during the period following World War II.

Drinking and the Postwar Campus

Concerns about undergraduate alcohol use dated back to the early twentieth century, but the 1940s saw a new approach to the problem. During the early twentieth century, many college administrators and mental hygiene experts advocated total abstinence and supported the temperance movement in the belief that it would eliminate the source of most undergraduate behavioral problems.[49] At Dartmouth, President Hopkins hailed the arrival of New Hampshire's tighter alcohol restrictions. While he didn't believe "alcohol ever did me any particular harm, and I enjoyed a certain use of it as much as most men I think," his observations on the close link between alcohol and "immorality" among Dartmouth students made him "unwilling any longer to become a patron of the liquor traffic even on a small scale." Instead, he believed that alcohol "ought to be put on the same basis as drugs and poisons of other kinds."[50]

After Prohibition ended in 1933, alcohol educators continued to stress a policy of total abstinence for adolescents and young adults even as moderate drinking became a normative part of postwar adult sociability.[51] The modern alcoholism movement—symbolized by the founding of Alcoholics Anonymous in 1935—promoted a new "multifaceted approach" to the problem of alcoholism. Alcohol researchers at Yale Center for Alcohol Studies, through the National Committee for Education on Alcoholism, emphasized a "disease concept rather than abstinence" and advocated "reform of the individual problem drinker through institutional care rather than through the nationwide prohibition of alcohol." In 1952, the APA classified alcoholism as a personality disorder in its first *Diagnostic and Statistical Manual* based on the psychodynamic perspective, which defined alcoholism as a sign of the individual's inability to adapt to his or her environment.[52]

Researchers at the Yale Center for Alcohol Studies became interested in the issue of college drinking in the late 1940s as a result of their close work with the University Health Service's Mental Hygiene Division. Fry regularly invited scientists from the center to hold staff workshops at which participants discussed the boundary between "normal" undergraduate social drinking and alcohol abuse. Fry, like other college mental hygienists at this time, observed that "drinking is an accepted symbol of good fellowship and an important part of the customs in many colleges." Popular singer Rudy Vallee had made Yale's "Whiffenpoof Song" and the University of Maine's "Stein Song" into national hits. Yet despite the ubiquity of alcohol on campus, Fry stated, only a "small percentage" of the students were "problem drinkers." In general, he found that excessive drinking and boisterous behavior were held in check by group standards. The extreme intoxication seen at some social and athletic events was usually "episodic, their frequency and duration being well controlled by a firm and sometimes indignant dean." According to Fry, heavy drinking was usually a form of compensation for those who could or would not fit in with their peers. "Immature" boys and girls, he observed, "may assign to drinking a false importance," while lonely students or those on the "social fringe" may "turn to the inns and drinking spots for their social life."[53]

Dr. Selden Bacon and Dr. Robert Straus of the Center for Alcohol Studies observed by the late 1940s that student deaths from drinking were on the rise and public interest in student drinking was increasing. Yet, they noted, "counseling students about the effects of alcohol in later life is not too effective because it is difficult for a young person to relate himself to a '45-year-old Skid Row' character." Concluding that "the hindrance to teaching objectively about alcoholism is that little is known about its development," they began a study of drinking customs and attitudes of college students, believed to be at the age when drinking started for most people.[54]

As soon as news of the study was released in March 1949, researchers came up against the prevalent popular assumption that "many students drink, that most of these drink frequently and to excess, and that the result is usually intoxication, often leading to situations involving serious problems, embarrassment, or disgrace." Coverage of the survey in the popular press made light of the work, joking, "Yale will get its facts about student drinking 'At a table down at Mory's,'" a New Haven bar popular among undergraduates. Four of the colleges the researchers approached declined to be interviewed because of fears that the "survey might lead to undesirable publicity" or because of campus policies of strict abstinence. The researchers also faced constant questions about their personal drinking practices from those who "found it inconceivable" that Straus and Bacon refused to take sides in the wet-dry controversy.[55]

The study covered twenty-seven colleges around the country, encompassing both public and private, coeducational and single-sex, white and black, nonsectarian and religious (including Catholic, Jewish, and Mormon colleges), and different regions of the country. The results were encouraging: Bacon and Straus found that "alcoholism is not a significant problem in the college population," largely because "alcoholism is a progressive disorder which, particularly in males, usually takes from 10 to 20 years to develop." They also noted that "for the great majority of college students drinking does not start in college, does not take place within the college, and shows no dominant collegiate pattern." More than half of the students reported that they had adopted the custom of drinking before age seventeen, and "the fact of being in college appears to have little influence on this behavior." Rather, drinking was part of the process of growing up for all adults, not just college students: "The armed forces, employers of late adolescents and the community itself face almost the same problems in relation to drinking among those of this age group as do the colleges." In short, college students were "not unlike most of the rest of the drinking population," and colleges "cannot realistically be asked to move faster than other institutions in the community and society" in dealing with drinking on campus. "The major contribution of the colleges, however, is to be made in the sphere of education," they declared. This meant discarding the Victorian tradition of total abstinence. They pointed out that the "majority of adults in our society do use alcoholic beverages, and ignorance or misinformation about the subject on the part of user or nonuser has nothing to commend it." Rather than attempting to reinforce an "old morality" or scare students to death by emphasizing the "most extreme pathologic manifestation of drinking," Bacon and Straus argued that colleges "should provide tested knowledge and intellectual training so that their students may meet this aspect of life with greater confidence and more understanding" by making responsible, adult decisions regarding alcohol consumption.[56]

Student Sexuality and the Pressures of Growing Up

Psychiatrists and deans alike found that alcohol use was intertwined with and often contributed to other problematic behaviors on campus, especially those associated with sexuality. Alfred Kinsey's best-selling studies of human sexual behavior indicated that extramarital sexual activity was becoming ever more common on the college campus and that homosexuality was far more prevalent than previously believed.[57] Straus and Bacon found that alcohol reduced inhibitions, and "of all the inhibitions imposed on individuals by our society, those in the sphere of sexual activity are among the strongest." They found that with both alcohol and sex, a "double standard" existed, allowing a "greater freedom of action to men than to women." Discussions with both male and female students found the "common belief that girls who drink may appear to be more popular with men but often are not taken seriously or respected: one can have a good time with a girl who drinks but may not consider her as a future wife." Women who were "regular" drinkers—defined as those who had drunk at least three times within the previous two weeks—had more dates with men "but were not nearly as apt to be 'engaged, pinned, or going steady with a young man.'"[58]

As with alcohol education, the key was instructing young people in mature, responsible attitudes toward the opposite sex. According to Fry, the most prominent elements that complicated the "whole process of growing up" included the "sexual development of the individual": nearly 40 percent of the problems he saw involved sex difficulties. These problems "were not for the most part problems of promiscuity or abnormal behavior." Rather, most students were confused and "lacked any realistic understanding of sex." This ignorance perpetuated sexual immaturity, he said, "and it is not surprising that those students who were immature sexually were immature in other ways as well."[59]

The most severe sign of sexual immaturity, said Fry, was homosexuality. According to Fry, "The majority of heavy drinkers were the homosexual type of person, who uses alcohol as a means of seduction. In addition, certain homosexuals faced with heterosexual experience will drink to evade the issue as a protection against sex."[60] Other psychiatrists found that "homosexual panic" or "uncontrollable perverse sexual cravings" were common sources of depression and anxiety among male college students, particularly those at single-sex institutions. According to Henry Harper Hart at Yale, it was unclear whether "casual companionship with girls in co-educational colleges reduces the incidence of homosexuality." Yet he noted that the modern men's college was "far from being the ascetic monastery from which it sprang. The opportunities for wholesome heterosexual experience are increasing, and do not appear to be inimical to good scholarship," he observed. "When sex becomes less and less an object of dread, guilt and shame," Hart concluded, "fears connected with it will diminish."[61]

Making sure that heterosexual experience remained "wholesome" was becoming increasingly problematic, however. Dean Everett Hunt of Swarthmore College, for example, observed at a 1953 symposium on "The Dean and the Psychiatrist" that his students regularly asked him if he had read the Kinsey report and what he thought of it. "They ask why the institution of chaperonage should be continued when it is so easily and constantly escaped." Students also inquired "why should not college men and women be given the wisest possible instruction as to dating and mating, and then be left to take care of their own relationships, with a recognition of their right to be alone when they please?"[62]

The answer at Swarthmore and elsewhere was to continue to enforce an elaborate system of parietal regulations. The sexual double standard ensured that parietals were not imposed on men, who were free to leave campus for sexual enjoyment. Yet in the interest of cultivating "qualities of maturity and responsibility in youth," skills considered essential to students' future roles as citizens in a democratic nation, administrators increasingly turned responsibility for enforcing these rules over to students themselves.[63] By the early 1950s, college physicians argued that fostering social and emotional maturity also meant involving students in the planning and organization of health services.

Mental Health Is Everybody's Business

In his opening address to the Fourth National Conference on Health in Colleges (1954), Farnsworth declared, "Times are changing and health programs must change with them." This meant addressing "not merely physical health but total health," giving equal weight to both mental and physical factors. "Although this point of view is not shared by all workers in this field," he admitted, "I am firmly convinced that mental health is everybody's business and that mental health is necessary in order to enable the college to carry on its chief function, namely, the dissemination of learning and addition of new knowledge." Farnsworth observed that "there has been comparatively little participation by students in the planning and organization of their own health services in this country," although "steps are being taken in this direction" at Stanford University. This trend was important not only to college health but to the nation's health more generally. "The more students can be encouraged to take part in the planning of health service functions," he argued, "the more likely they are to be intelligent leaders and planners in community health matters at a later period."[64]

Students from the U.S. National Student Association helped plan this conference, and they other student leaders expressed their opinions at a session on student participation. According to the conference report, the discussion constituted a "lively demonstration of student participation in action." That students who attended "felt free to criticize and question their elders was in itself an indication of the freedom to which they had grown accustomed in their own institutions. In their manner and their intelligent participation, one saw reflected their own steady march toward the goal of higher education," which the professionals who attended the conference agreed was the "preparation of the student for his place in and contribution to the adult society of which he will become a part." While "adolescent high spirits, the need to rebel, and other disturbing characteristics of the young will intrude in this process," they observed, "responsibility for oneself and towards one's fellows will grow as the student begins to derive satisfaction from it and comes to have an understanding of its broader implications."[65] This new commitment to a truly "student-centered" health service that allowed students an unprecedented role in health care planning, would have unintended consequences in the ensuing decade.

CHAPTER 7

Student Bodies and Student Rights

During the early morning hours of 30 April 1968, a thousand New York City policemen stormed five Columbia University buildings occupied by demonstrating students and faculty. The police action was the culmination of several months of protests at the university against the presence of military and Central Intelligence Agency recruiters on campus as well as the proposed construction of a new gymnasium in a public park on Morningside Heights. Many students saw the new gymnasium, intended primarily to improve the athletic facilities for male undergraduates, as a symbol of the Ivy League institution's elitism and racism. The 30 April conflict between police and protesters lasted for three hours, during which students and faculty were thrown or dragged down stairs, pulled by their hair, punched, kicked, and bloodied. "A diabetic student fell into a coma," reported an article in the *Nation*. "One faculty member suffered a nervous collapse. Many students bled profusely from head wounds opened by handcuffs wielded as weapons. Dozens of moaning people lay about the grass unattended."[1]

By the early 1970s, similar scenes had been duplicated across the country. Beginning on 1 February 1960, when four black students at North Carolina Agricultural and Technical College sat at a whites-only lunch counter in Greensboro, refusing to leave until they received service, growing numbers of young men and women put their bodies and lives in jeopardy in support of civil rights, disarmament, free speech, feminism, and an end to the war in Vietnam. Others demanded new rights to enjoy their bodies free from administrative scrutiny and traditional forms of morality. At Columbia, for example, undergraduates formed the Columbia University Sexual Freedom Forum in response to the institution's crackdown on parietal rules in the early 1960s. One male senior wrote in an editorial in the student newspaper, "If girls are kept out of the rooms by college edict, the students will, as alumni, withhold financial support from the university."[2] At Vassar College, students were outraged when President Sarah Gibson Blanding warned in a 1962 lecture that drunkenness and "sexual experimentation" were considered "indecent" behavior and grounds for expulsion from the college. "What I do in private and discreetly is entirely my personal concern," wrote one student to the *Vassar Miscellany News*, adding that when she applied, she had been under the impression the college's faith in liberal education included respect for the students' intelligence and ability to make informed, mature decisions. "If Vassar is to become the Poughkeepsie Victorian Seminary for Young Virgins, then the change of policy had better be made explicit in admissions catalogues," she declared.[3]

Physicians on college campuses became accustomed to treating students injured during protests as well as to fielding increasing requests for advice on birth control, sexuality, and the use of illegal drugs. According to Harvard health services director Dana Farnsworth, he and other college physicians were surprised by the intensity of student dissatisfaction with campus life. Although periodic student protest against allegedly "repressive" administrative policies had occurred since the beginning of higher education, Farnsworth observed, the "widespread suspicion and hostility" among students during the 1960s constituted a "relatively new phenomenon."[4]

As in the 1950s, college psychiatrists found themselves trying to interpret the causes of campus unrest. Some psychiatrists explained incidents of student protest much the same way they had the previous decade—that is, as extreme signs of adolescent maladjustment. Farnsworth, for example, observed in 1964, "The gap between intellectual and emotional maturity in late adolescence is getting wider." He added, "Many of the most exceptional students are among the most immature." Dr. Sutherland Miller Jr., director of counseling at Columbia, blamed the problem on parents who were preoccupied with personal success and faculty who were "too busy with research and 'productivity.'" He observed that prolonged education also expanded the period of adolescence, with the "crutches" of family economic and emotional support making the young enter the adult world with "little sense of responsibility or the ability to withstand stress." Experts at both Harvard and Columbia concluded that students "lack a sense of security because neither the home nor the college defines explicitly the limits of permissiveness." Both psychiatrists and deans saw the answer as "less permissiveness," even if it led to more student protests. The role of campus psychiatrists was to counsel the "less-than-ill—before their malaise becomes a malady" and to help colleges "establish academically productive rules, life and setting."[5]

A younger cohort of psychiatrists and physicians, some of whom had worked closely with students on the front lines of various social movements of the decade, increasingly challenged this view. The most notable members of this new group of progressive physicians included Robert Coles, a research psychiatrist from the Harvard University health service, and Joseph Brenner, a physician from the Massachusetts Institute of Technology health service, who served as medical staff for the Mississippi Summer Project in 1964. Coles and Brenner evaluated applicants for the project and provided medical and psychiatric advice during the orientation sessions at Western College for Women in Oxford, Ohio. During the applicant interviews, Coles and Brenner soon realized the volunteers were no different than the students they saw in their regular practices. Far from being "psychopathic" or "immature," the students they saw "were almost uniformly intelligent, determined youth, willfully desirous of ending what to most of them was a deeply felt sense of injustice in their country." While in the field in Mississippi, Coles and Brenner studied how students responded to a "rather trying and even dangerous summer" that included hundreds of "arrests, jailings, bombings, shootings, beatings and threats." Although some students succumbed to various "war neuroses" caused by the "near battle-like situations," their consciences, compassion, and commitment to the work as well the "group spirit" kept most of the students psychologically healthy. Coles and Brenner concluded, "There is a specific role for psychiatrists, psychologists, and social workers in the civil rights struggle," but this role "requires a respectful willingness on the part of the professional. These are not 'sick' people; nor is their struggle in its essence anything but part of our common need for the dignity of all men."[6]

This desire for "human dignity" continued when students returned to their campuses, where they became increasingly dissatisfied with restrictions on speech and behavior they believed were out of step with democratic principles. Drawing on the language of the civil rights movement, students attacked the "institutionalized paternalism" restricting their on-campus freedoms, much in the same way that other activists had attacked institutionalized racism and sexism.

Sex and the College Student in the 1960s

Nowhere was this demand for personal freedom more apparent than in the escalating conflict over student sexual behavior in the early 1960s. Indeed, students often framed their demands for equality in explicitly sexual terms. At the University of California at Berkeley, one of the founders of the Free Speech Movement, Mario Salvo, described the university's rules restricting political activity on and near campus as "emasculation or attempted emasculation."[7]

Similar movements occurred on other campuses, prompting the Committee on the College Student of the Group for the Advancement of Psychiatry (GAP) to investigate parietals at both single-sex and coeducational schools. One of the key collaborators on the GAP report was Robert L. Arnstein, who became director of Yale's Mental Hygiene Division in 1961. The year before, the university had seen a sex scandal in which twenty students were arrested and fined for having "lascivious carriage" (sexual acts not involving intercourse) with a fourteen-year-old girl from nearby Hamden. Twelve of the students resigned from the university, and the other eight were expelled.[8] Arnstein recalled that when he began at the health service, "birth control issues were paramount, and fear of pregnancy was a real source of anxiety," not just for women but for men as well. For Yale students, the "major responsibility for the prevention of pregnancy was the male's" as a consequence of Connecticut state law prohibiting the sale or distribution of all contraceptives except condoms (which were exempted in the larger interest of preventing the spread of venereal disease), even to married couples. Thus, condoms were the main method of birth control, "and withdrawal was a frequently used, if rather uncertain, contraceptive practice." Yale students frequently visited the mental health service with acute anxiety about the possibility that they had impregnated their sexual partners. Arnstein also observed that for male students, "lack of sexual experience" was a frequent source of psychological distress. "It was not uncommon for a male student to come for therapy and confess that he was a virgin, implying he was the only one left on campus." Masturbation was also a "frequent source of anxiety, concern, and guilt," since published statements even by mental health professionals "remained ambiguous." Homosexuality too continued to be the "source of considerable guilt and unhappiness," although "its prevalence was difficult to estimate because it tended to be hidden and even in therapy sessions, spoken about with some hesitation."[9]

Homosexuality could also end a student's career at Yale, since the university had a zero-tolerance policy regarding this "perversion." After the student newspaper published a 1952 anti-coeducation article, "Keep Yale Homosexual," in which the author defended homosexuality as a noble practice "countenanced in early Greece," the Mental Hygiene Division decided to take harsh measures to stamp out homosexuality on campus. For especially intractable cases, Clement Fry believed he had to violate patient confidentiality to ensure that other students "are not raided by these homosexual tendencies or people responsible for these tendencies."[10]

Arnstein, however, was fully committed to student confidentiality. He recalled that in the early 1960s, he was "enthusiastic" about working on the GAP report because it would allow experiences to be pooled, thereby protecting the identity of particular students.[11] The 1965 report, *Sex and the College Student*, surveyed forty-nine institutions—small and large; urban, suburban, and rural; from the East, West, and Midwest. The report observed that "college students are asserting with increasing militancy their right to privacy and self-determination in matters pertaining to their own sexual activity." It noted that female students were especially strident in their demands for sexual freedom. "There is consensus that the double standard is increasingly being discarded and that college girls more often seek sexual experience during the college years than did their mothers." Students, both male and female, were especially vigilant in their demands for contraception: "Many college students view contraceptive information as a right that is due them" and were well informed about the various methods available, including the latest invention, the contraceptive pill. The report argued, "The student's privacy requires respect: sexual activity practiced with appropriate attention to the sensitivities of other people should not be the direct concern of the administration." Yet the report also cautioned, "In a dormitory situation, regulations are necessary to maintain order and to control behavior that impinges upon the freedom and privacy of other students." These regulations should be constructed to "encourage informal contacts but maintain some measure of available external control so that students will feel neither burdened nor frightened by their freedom."[12]

The notion of a right to privacy in sexual matters alluded to the Supreme Court's recent landmark decision, *Griswold v. Connecticut*, which found that "Connecticut's birth-control law unconstitutionally intrudes upon the right of marital privacy."[13] Not until 1972 did the Court extend the same right of privacy to the unmarried, however.[14] Until then, most states either remained silent on the issue of whether the unwed had the same privacy rights or explicitly outlawed prescribing or distributing contraceptives to unmarried individuals. Massachusetts and Wisconsin had the strictest contraceptive laws in the nation, as both continued to prohibit giving contraceptives to unmarried persons. Violation of these birth control laws was a felony carrying a punishment of up to five years in prison. Other states were less restrictive, but very few allowed unmarried individuals, especially those below the age of twenty-one, to obtain birth control without parental consent.[15]

Despite its respect for student privacy, the GAP report advised that dispensing contraceptives "cannot be done routinely or casually" and warned that "many students will interpret the dispensation of contraceptive devices as sanction for their use." Instead, the report's authors believed that dispensing contraceptive information was the most appropriate solution to student inquiries, since it would respect patient autonomy by placing responsibility for using this information in the student's hands.[16]

The Contraceptive Revolution on Campus

Getting one's hands on contraceptives depended on a mixture of persistence, ingenuity, and above all location, since most states outlawed the distribution of contraceptives to unwed minors. Physicians who violated state laws risked loss of the licenses and/or prison. Dr. Roswell Johnson, director of the health service at Brown University, was arrested and jailed in 1965 for violating Rhode Island state law by prescribing pills to unmarried Pembroke students. Johnson's practices were revealed by a reporter for the *Pembroke Recorder* for whom Johnson had refused to prescribe the pill because she was below the age of twenty-one. However, he considered anyone who had reached the age of majority a "free agent." Johnson argued that he was "not contributing to unmitigated promiscuity" but rather was "contributing to a solid relationship" by preventing pregnancies among the unwed.[17] Although Johnson stated that his actions were "simply my own private orientation" and did not represent university policy, Brown President Barnaby C. Keeny supported the health director, stating that Johnson's appointment as university physician gave him "broad discretion to treat cases as seems best to him in light of his knowledge and judgment." However, Brown officials reaffirmed that unwed minors could not expect the same services and pointed out that Johnson treated women engaged to be married who were referred to the health service by the campus ministry.[18]

Even Brown's limited birth control policy was unusual. Officials at Columbia, the University of Pennsylvania, the University of California, and the University of Michigan, among others, told *Newsweek* magazine in 1965 that they did not intend to offer contraceptive services. The few who did prescribe the pill, such as physicians at Stanford, Illinois, and Minnesota, stated that they would do so only to those who were already married or showed "bona fide intent" to get married. At Bennington College, health director Dorothy Hager believed that birth control was the responsibility of private doctors, adding that she did not feel it was her duty to "either pierce ears or to prescribe premarital contraceptives, devices, or medication." The University of Chicago was more liberal: there, health service director Richard H. Moy argued that since contraception was "strictly a medical decision," a woman could get the pill if the service thought it "appropriate." Yet unmarried women were required to consult with the psychiatric service before they could receive prescriptions.[19] Officials at most institutions believed that providing contraception or even advice about birth control would lead to a further decline in campus morals. According to a 1966 survey conducted by the ACHA, physicians at only thirteen U.S. colleges and universities prescribed oral contraceptives to unmarried students, and most of these did so only for women over the age of twenty-one.[20]

In Massachusetts, officials at most public and private institutions of higher education stated that they did not intend to follow Brown's example. At Harvard, Farnsworth said that the "supervision of contraceptive practices of unmarried students is not an appropriate function in a college health service." Boston University's student health director, Samuel E. Leard, said, "We do not condone this thing at all. It's morally wrong and here in Massachusetts it's against the law." Officials at Smith, Simmons, Emerson, and Northeastern made similar comments.[21]

One exception was Dr. Robert Gage at the University of Massachusetts, who provided diaphragms and birth control pills to undergraduate and graduate women with full administrative approval despite state law prohibiting this practice. Gage recalled, "We were treading on pretty thin ice," by prescribing birth control to unmarried women. "Matter of fact, you wondered if there was any ice there at all," given the Commonwealth's restrictive contraceptive laws. Nevertheless, Gage realized, "something had to be done" to address the needs of students who "had had enough" of in loco parentis. "We felt we had to treat young people as adults who were able to make their own decisions."[22]

It would not be long before someone would step forward to overtly test Massachusetts's birth control laws. In the spring of 1967, students at Boston University contacted thirty-four-year-old medical school dropout and contraceptive salesman William R. Baird about the possibility of giving a lecture for students at BU and other area colleges. Baird had already gained notoriety in his home state of New York, where he had been arrested for operating a birth control clinic in Hempstead, Long Island, and using a mobile "plan van" to disseminate birth control information and free equipment in poor neighborhoods.[23] Baird's allies in his birth control "crusade" included a group of students at Hofstra University, also in Hempstead, who frequently turned to Baird for contraceptive advice. As Baird told *Ramparts*, a liberal Catholic alternative newspaper, he was "surprised how naïve about sex some of those bright college kids are," since ignorance was the main reason so many wound up at his clinic seeking abortions.[24] Hofstra students also served as volunteers for Baird's Parents' Aid Society. These students, led by Douglas Wilcox, soon formed the Parents' Aid Club, the first birth control organization for students on a college campus that enjoyed the blessings of both the administration and the student government. "I think it's a good thing for them to do," said Dean of Students Randall Hoffman. "Students need this kind of information and don't ordinarily get it—either at home or from us."[25]

Young people in greater Boston proved just as eager for Baird's message. On 6 April 1967, Baird spoke to more than twenty-five hundred people, most of them students, at Boston University's Hayden Hall. Even students from nearby Boston College, a Catholic institution, "successfully defied threats from the college's dean and turned out in force to listen to Baird's talk." During the lecture, Baird displayed various contraceptives and gave an unmarried female student a can of Emko contraceptive foam. After the lecture ended, the Boston vice squad arrested Baird and charged him with "crimes against chastity."[26] Two years later, Baird was again arrested after a demonstration at Northland College in Ashland, Wisconsin.[27] Baird won the support of other college students throughout the nation, who formed the nucleus of the group picketing for Baird's release.[28]

While Baird's appeals worked their way through the court system, students took matters into their own hands by creating advice manuals and student-led sex education classes. At BU, the Student Congress published a "handy guide" on birth control, abortion, and venereal disease as an "act of civil disobedience" against the Boston police. These students, most of them women, worked closely with feminist organizations in Boston and Cambridge and held public demonstrations defending Baird and demanding reproductive rights for women.[29] At nearby Radcliffe College, students complained that when they went to the college health service for contraceptive advice and other "female problems, they were made to feel guilty or abnormal."[30] To meet the need for accurate knowledge, students put together a guide to birth control providers in the Boston area that served as a model for the feminist classic, *Our Bodies, Ourselves.*[31] During the late 1960s and early 1970s, dozens of other advice manuals appeared on campuses throughout the country with such flippant titles as *Between Your Navel and Your Knees* (University of Houston); *Everything You Always Wanted to Know about Birth Control but Were Afraid to Ask* (Colorado State University); and *How to Have Intercourse without Getting Screwed* (University of Washington).[32]

Male students played an important role in this contraceptive "self-help" movement. James Trussell, an undergraduate at all-male Davidson College outside Charlotte, North Carolina, began offering lectures on birth control to his classmates during the late 1960s. Trussell first became interested in population issues as a high school student in Columbus, Georgia, where "I saw some of my classmates drop out because of [unplanned pregnancies], and I began to think of how stupid and sad it was that high school students don't know about birth control." Trussell was soon asked to expand his lectures to include women students at nearby Queens College under a program called Free University sponsored by student groups at both Davidson and Queens. Trussell recalled, "There were quite a few girls in my course, some out of curiosity, I think. I suppose some of them were embarrassed at times, but no one was pushed to say anything. There was no forcing."[33] In the summer of 1970, Trussell received a grant from the Institute for the Study of Health and Society, developed by the moderate student group Students of the American Medical Association to give future medical professionals experience working among nonelite populations and in remote areas. In the introduction to *The Loving Book*, an advice manual resulting from Trussell's work with the institute, Trussell and coauthor Steve Chandler wrote, "We are both college students who have seen the very real need for this type of information in our own schools and communities. It is hoped that those who read this manual will gain a greater insight into their own sexuality."[34]

In response to student activism, some physicians openly argued that campus health centers should ignore state laws regarding the treatment of unmarried women. Yale University started offering contraceptive and sex counseling services to students shortly after going coed in 1969, even though the *Griswold* decision applied only to married women. "When Yale first started admitting women undergraduates," said Yale gynecologist Dr. Philip Sarrel, "the officials had fantasies that all the young girls descending on campus would get pregnant." To alleviate these fears, Yale hired Sarrel and his wife, Lorna, a psychiatric social worker, to set up a counseling service to provide not only contraceptives but sex education and relationship advice as well.[35] Sarrel urged his colleagues at other institutions not to "hide behind the law," declaring, "If it is good medical practice to prevent a girl from becoming pregnant"—and he believed that such was the case for many young, unmarried women—"then the law should be circumvented so that the girl does not go to a criminal abortionist."[36] Marguerite Shearer, staff gynecologist at the University of Michigan, likewise informed the *Detroit Free Press* that she would continue to prescribe contraceptives to female students, regardless of marital status, adding, "Morality based on fear is no morality at all." When the university regents considered "pulling the pill out of the student health clinic," Shearer said, "'They can have my job in a hand basket,' if she, as doctor at the University health service could not practice medicine as she saw fit."[37] At Harvard, pressure from students became so great that in 1971, the health service hired a full-time gynecologist and coordinated gynecological services, sex counseling, and abortion referrals. According to Radcliffe president Mary Ingraham Bunting, the health service should take an "'educational' responsibility in the field of sexuality."[38]

Even a few Catholic institutions permitted students to learn about birth control, although these schools stopped short of allowing contraceptives to be distributed on campus. Undergraduate women at Thomas More College, a division of Roman Catholic Fordham University in the Bronx, successfully petitioned the administration to add courses on birth control to the curriculum in 1967. One of the students who presented the petition to the administration, Victoria Perrulli, stated that the request had been made because the students felt that "without real information on birth control, there is no way to make a personal decision." Perrulli added she and other students were not asking the college to dispense contraceptives, but "we feel there should be more information on birth control and contraceptive devices while we are still in college." The dean of students, Dr. Martin J. Meade, gave them his full support, stating that he believed it appropriate for any qualified member of the university health service staff to give accurate information on birth control. In fact, he saw this information as a natural extension of existing courses on marriage and the family.[39]

These cases were still relatively rare. A 1970 ACHA survey indicated that the number of institutions offering contraceptive services had increased to 118, but this represented a small percentage of the more than 2,500 U.S. colleges and universities at that time. Although schools did not state their reasons for not offering birth control, fear of prosecution probably played a role.[40] Another powerful disincentive was concern about the impact offering contraceptive services would have on state funding and alumni donations. As one recent graduate of Mills College in California sarcastically told *Glamour* magazine in 1970, "If Mills came out strong for birth control, some little old lady in Menlo Park might decide this is just a bit much from her old alma mater and withhold her yearly check."[41]

Students who could not find birth control on campus resorted to services in the local community. At the University of North Carolina, Chapel Hill, students sought the advice of Dr. Takey Crist, a gynecologist at North Carolina Memorial Hospital and a member of the faculty in the UNC School of Medicine's Department of Obstetrics and Gynecology. Crist recalled that while he was an intern in Charleston, South Carolina, he had helped care for a nineteen-year-old African American student who needed a total hysterectomy following a botched illegal abortion. Crist believed that it was unfair that female undergraduates who became pregnant were expelled for "unwomanly conduct" while male students went unpunished. When he went to UNC to do his residency, Crist began visiting sororities, dormitories, and student organizations to give lectures on contraception and prevention of sexually transmitted diseases.[42] Crist and undergraduate Lana Starnes also started a sex information column in the campus newspaper, the *Daily Tar Heel*, in which they answered questions regarding sex and contraception as well as more routine hygiene questions such as whether an unmarried girl should use tampons or sanitary napkins. Crist called on other campuses to do the same, arguing, "It is not our job to establish what is good or bad, but what is necessary."[43]

The Planned Parenthood College Program

Elsewhere, students found local Planned Parenthood affiliates especially helpful in offering access to reliable birth control. *Time* magazine reported in 1969 that at Stanford, many of the university's "2,820 coeds are now seeking contraceptive help at the nearby Palo Alto Planned Parenthood center." In fact, the center's director, Gloria Davis, complained that the clinic could barely accommodate the crowds of students.[44] At the University of California at Berkeley, the staff was willing to make birth control information but not contraceptives available to students. In 1967, one of the staff psychiatrists, Dr. Eugene Schoenfeld, started a column, "Doctor Hip Pocrates," in the *Berkeley Barb*, an alternative newspaper. The column answered questions about sex, birth control, psychoactive drugs, and other controversial health issues in a low-key, nonjudgmental, often humorous manner. Other alternative and college newspapers soon picked up the column, and its advice was eventually collected in a best-selling book, *Doctor Hip Pocrates: Advice Your Family Doctor Never Gave You* (1969).[45]

Yet UC health services director Dr. Henry Bruyn did not think the health service bore responsibility for prescribing or distributing contraceptive pills or devices.[46] Consequently, Planned Parenthood of Alameda County in nearby Oakland found that Berkeley students comprised 60 percent of its caseload.[47] When Sam Sloan, president of the Sexual Freedom League, confronted assistant health service director Dr. Gertrude Mitchell with these facts as well as the observation that many young women without cars found the Oakland clinic inaccessible, Mitchell replied they could take the bus. Furthermore, she stated, "The pill isn't the answer," since most college women were too immature and irresponsible to handle sex or contraception. Instead, Mitchell declared, "I will stand by the method approved by the Catholic Church, your grandmother, and everybody else: total abstinence."[48]

In response to student interest regarding birth control at Berkeley and elsewhere, Planned Parenthood–World Population initiated its Program of Student Community Action in 1969, appointing twenty-five-year-old Dan Pellegrom as its director. Pellegrom was a recent graduate of Columbia University, where he had served as Student Council president during the student strike of 1968. Pellegrom and other Planned Parenthood officials were heartened by the enthusiasm of college students and tried to cultivate a relationship that would encourage a "free exchange of ideas" by responding to student initiatives rather than dictating to them.[49] The organization also used popular culture icons such as Joan Baez to attract students to the college program.[50] The program also drew on broader concerns about the "population explosion," although Pellegrom and other leaders intended to expand population concerns beyond the traditional focus on impoverished minorities in the United States and the developing world.[51] Planned Parenthood leaders hoped that a college program would not only "acquaint college students with the latest contraceptive techniques and devices and provide them with information about availability and accessibility" and "provide a vehicle" for establishing contraceptive services on college campuses but also "motivate college students to have smaller families through the voluntary use of the latest, most effective, and safest contraceptive methods."[52]

Officials at Planned Parenthood–World Population acknowledged that many students supported the birth control movement because of concerns about the impact of overpopulation on the environment. These officials therefore actively reached out to the Sierra Club and other environmental groups that were beginning to appear on college campuses.[53] The first U.S. Earth Day celebration, held in 1970, "made U.S. population limitation a major theme." The group Zero Population Growth (ZPG), founded by biologists concerned about the "catastrophic impacts of ever more human beings on the biosphere," sponsored "teach-ins" for college students in April 1969, leading to the creation of dozens of ZPG college chapters around the country.[54] Several self-help books that appeared on colleges were prompted by ecological concerns. For example, during Earth Week in April 1970, students at Duke University compiled and distributed *A Guide to Contraception and Abortion.* The UNC publication *Elephants and Butterflies* was likewise sponsored in part by the student conservation group ECOS, and ecology groups at other campuses soon followed this example.[55]

Yet the alliance between birth control advocates and the population movement was an uneasy one. Officials at the Planned Parenthood Federation of America were especially cautious about ZPG's appeal on college campuses. Pellegrom told University of Connecticut biology professor Nancy Clark that given the controversial nature of ZPG and population groups more generally, it was "essential" that Planned Parenthood provide leadership at the ZPG's teach-ins and use it as a way to increase student interest in forming campus Planned Parenthood chapters. Pellegrom warned of the dangers of affiliating with ZPG, however. Based on his experience working with black community groups, he had "personal problems" with ZPG, "one, because their rhetoric could be taken by the black communities as genocidal and two, because they seem to be often politically inept."[56] Pellegrom added that although many students were eager to create campus affiliates and often shared Pellegrom's uneasiness with the term *zero-population growth*, they found the term *planned parenthood* outdated and irrelevant to those who had no intention of becoming parents in the foreseeable future. Instead, some students suggested using "Freedom to

Understand Contraceptive Knowledge," the initials of which made an "attractive title for college students."[57]

This increasingly strained relationship between Planned Parenthood leaders and the population movement did not prevent the college program from raising the fury of a few African American leaders. In the fall of 1969, Louis Lomax, a black studies professor at Hofstra, alleged that two nineteen-year-old black students had been put in a clinical trial of low-estrogen birth control pills. Some black students had also complained to Lomax about "Planned Parenthood's aggressive recruitment program on the campus." In response, Planned Parenthood–World Population affiliates director Naomi Gray, also an African American, agreed to meet with Lomax and other black faculty to discuss the problem.[58]

The results of this meeting are unknown, as is the point of view of the black women at Hofstra. Elsewhere, however, many black female students were at least as adamant as their white counterparts in seeking access to birth control. One study of four thousand college women, white and black, attending coeducational and single-sex institutions in the southeastern United States found that "these young members of the educational elite expect the physician to provide contraceptive information. They are especially interested in hearing from him about 'the pill.'"[59] Planned Parenthood leaders recognized that enlisting the black students' support was essential in establishing the legitimacy of birth control within the African American community both on and off campus. Douglas Stewart, director of Planned Parenthood's Office of Community Relations and an African American, said that "birth control programs might fare better" if more blacks served in local Planned Parenthood affiliates, and having a significant black presence in the organization on both the local and national level would go a long way toward counteracting charges of "genocide," which left "so many people caught between pressures from militant groups and their own wishes for fewer children."[60] Therefore, the college program eagerly encouraged participation by African American students, and one of the earliest college chapters was at the historically black Hampton Institute in Virginia.

White students also challenged the racist assumptions of the more extreme population control advocates. Trussell, for example, said that his experience working with impoverished blacks in the Muscogee County, Georgia, health department family planning clinics led him to remark, "When all the programs are aimed toward the poor blacks, it's not difficult to understand why some of them think that family planning is an attempt at genocide." He added, "There just aren't enough poor people to cause that big of a population problem. . . . [T]hese programs have to reach the middle class as well, and every college student should be aware of the fact that his third child is going to expand the problem."[61]

At the other end of the political spectrum, Planned Parenthood officials expressed some qualms about what they considered to be the more extreme student organizations, particularly those representing radical feminist positions on the "medical establishment." For example, Planned Parenthood–World Population president Alan F. Guttmacher and college program director Gene Vadies were ambivalent about the *Birth Control Handbook*, produced by students at McGill University in Montreal. The authors of the McGill handbook proclaimed that their manual had been "produced not as a favor to an irresponsible medical profession nor as a favor to men who want an easy but 'safe' lay, but as a political act. Organizations distributing the Handbook have a responsibility to continually raise the issues of women's liberation whenever dealing with birth control."[62] In their speech to the ACHA, Guttmacher and Vadies called the McGill handbook an "excellent effort seriously tarnished by mixing leftist political opinions with sex information." As more sensible models, they pointed to "nonpolitical" brochures such as *Elephants and Butterflies* from the University of North Carolina. They also suggested that physicians should help students come up with less controversial titles, observing the University of Washington's *How to Have Intercourse without Getting Screwed* offended "some of the more conservative faculty members of that university," who "registered objections to the title, not to the contents."[63]

Planned Parenthood also remained adamant that contraception should be distributed only by trained medical professionals and hoped to use student activism to pressure campus health centers to provide reproductive services to students. In a 1970 interview with *Glamour* magazine, Pellegrom said, "Students don't realize their own lobbying strength: They should push for campus birth-control clinics now—while health services are trying to reconsider their Victorian policies." As a preliminary tactic, Pellegrom advised students to force their universities to take a stand on establishing a clinic, acknowledging that most positions would probably be negative—for example, "The college doesn't want to contribute to declining morals." Pellegrom also advised students to take the position that "by denying the health-service doctor the right to dispense contraceptives, [the administration] is interfering with the doctor-patient relationship; then, you can pressure your health service to get going and set up a clinic or at least an open referral policy to direct girls to private doctors."[64]

For such campus campaigns to succeed, Planned Parenthood officials realized that they also had to convert college health care professionals to the cause. In a speech at the 1972 annual meeting of the ACHA, Guttmacher and Vadies pointed to charges that the "new sexual morality" of college students was "far ahead of the medical profession." They asked rhetorically whether the proliferation of student-written pamphlets and student-led sex counseling groups constituted an "indictment of the inadequacy in this area of college health services? We do not know," Guttmacher and Vadies admitted, "but more than likely the students fear judgmental attitudes and moralizing by their elders, neither of which they receive from peers." They concluded their speech by asking the ACHA and Planned Parenthood–World Population to work together, pleading with "those who still have them to slough their prejudices and hangups" and "face sex on the campus with realism and tolerant understanding. Help students introduce a broad-based course on human sexuality and, above all, see that humane, easily obtainable sexual counseling, including contraceptive service, is readily available to all students who seek it irrespective of age or marital status."[65] These efforts to establish reproductive health services on campus were greatly aided by the U.S. Supreme Court's *Eisenstadt v. Baird* decision: "If the right of privacy means anything, it is the right of the individual, married or single, to be free from unwarranted governmental intrusion into matters so fundamentally affecting a person as the decision whether to bear or beget a child."[66]

Birth control and reproductive health were not the only areas in which students asserted their right to privacy: the decade also saw increasing concerns about patient confidentiality more generally, especially in the area of mental health.

The Psychiatrist as Change Agent

In 1967, Thomas Szasz, a professor of psychiatry at Upstate Medical Center in Syracuse, New York, launched a scathing attack on what he considered the questionable ethics of college psychiatry. Szasz had "long maintained that the psychiatrist impersonates the medical role; actually, he is an interpreter of moral rules and an enforcer of social expectations and laws. This is especially true of the bureaucratic psychiatrist," he claimed, "that is, of the psychiatrist who is the paid agent of an institution rather than of an individual." By the late 1960s, Szasz had already gained a reputation as a maverick who denied the existence of mental illness and believed the profession of psychiatry threatened civil liberties. Szasz singled out Farnsworth and other Harvard psychiatrists for scorn, using their writings as evidence for his claim that the "college psychiatrist is a therapist in name only." In fact, said Szasz, "he is a double agent," serving both the students and the administration "but owing real loyalty to neither. Toward the students the college psychiatrist shows one side of his Janus-like face: He is a compassionate counselor and therapist who promises to be a faithful conspirator with the student in his struggle for liberation from parents and educational authorities." Yet "toward the institution and the outside world," Szasz claimed, "he shows the other side of his face: He is a wise physician who will select and control students and inform about them, as the needs of the school and community require."[67]

Like much of his writings, Szasz's charges against college psychiatry were exaggerated, but they did reflect the increasingly awkward role in which college psychiatrists found themselves by the late 1960s. It did not help the reputation of college psychiatry that Farnsworth was a harsh critic of the student movements, which he dismissed as "transient adolescent acting-out" caused by permissive postwar child-rearing advice. As he told the ACHA in 1969, "It is not the function of the psychiatrist to inform administration members of infractions of rules, but neither is it his job (nor is it therapeutic) to use his influence to rescue and by implication excuse a student from the consequences of his behavior." He concluded that health workers' primary responsibility was "to help any individual who is at odds with his environment, for whatever reason." For this reason, "the health service in particular should not become politicized for, if it avoids identification with one side or the other, it can be very helpful in facilitating communication between opposing groups such as radical students and more conservative faculty or administrative members."[68]

Farnsworth's counterpart at Yale found himself compelled to adopt the role of "change agent," looking beyond the unhappy state of the individual to aspects of the system that caused emotional problems. At Yale, one of the major issues was student demands for coeducation, as part of which a group of undergraduates asked Arnstein to make a statement in favor of admitting women to the college: "Their spokesman said, 'You must be for coeducation because you are for mental health.' In his mind," Arnstein recalled, "the two were clearly linked and I should be pushing for the change." In response, Arnstein said that he "was not sure their statement was correct," since there was "no evidence from coeducational campuses that the number [of psychiatric problems] was lower, although the problems might be different."[69]

Nevertheless, Arnstein felt obliged to change the mental hygiene department's policy regarding patient confidentiality. Under Fry, the department's official policy was to ask for written permission from the student before confidential information was released. Yet Fry felt no qualms about violating patient confidentiality "in the case of a homosexual applying for a position to tutor young boys, or where some true psychopathic personality would not fit into the position which the Bureau of Personnel had open." During the 1940s and 1950s, the Mental Hygiene Division also fielded requests from outside agencies, especially the Federal Bureau of Investigation, conducting investigations of applicants' backgrounds. Fry wrote to J. Edgar Hoover in 1950 that he had "seen many of your agents in the past" as well as "representatives from the armed forces regarding former patients." In cases of "subversive" activity—including homosexuality—Fry wrote, he "would not hesitate to give information." Arnstein found this statement "rather chilling" and worked to clarify the department's position on patient confidentiality when he assumed the directorship.[70] In 1964, Arnstein received a request from Dr. William Menninger and Dr. Joseph English for information on Peace Corps applicants. Arnstein replied, "Any policy we established had to apply for agencies other than the Peace Corps," noting that a student signing a waiver to release confidential information "was considerably less voluntary than suggested" when under the pressure of an application for a position with an outside agency, graduate school, or professional school. Furthermore, "knowledge that information might be available to outside agencies could cause students to decide against seeking therapy." At the same time, Arnstein received requests from male undergraduates who wanted psychiatric exemptions from military service in Vietnam. After "considerable thought," Arstein and his staff "decided to retain our policy and release no more information to draft boards than we would to the Peace Corps or anyone else."[71]

By the mid-1960s, some health care professionals were beginning to sense that students were shunning campus health services as a consequence of fears of confidentiality violations, especially when their problems involved reproductive health care, sexually transmitted diseases, and consumption of illegal drugs. Others were simply disgusted by the conservative attitudes of many college health care personnel. Farnsworth, for example, wrote that many students "are genuinely concerned over social injustices but are willing to exploit others and be totally parasitic on society." They also appeared "bent on shocking those with whom they disagree (mainly their parents and other members of the older generation) by their appearance, sexual customs, drug usage, disdain of work, and disregard of principles of sanitation."[72] Realizing that such attitudes prevented students from seeking medical care, liberal physicians began creating alternative services in the community to serve those who for whatever reason felt uncomfortable consulting campus health services.

Free Clinics

The first of these alternative services was the Haight-Ashbury Free Clinic, founded by David Smith and Richard Seymour in San Francisco in 1967 in response to the health needs of the thousands of young people who flocked to the city during the infamous Summer of Love. Although the majority of clientele were runaways and/or too poor to afford traditional health care services, Smith and Seymour also soon found themselves treating students from Berkeley, San Francisco State, and other area colleges and universities who were "turned off" by the condescending attitudes of conservative doctors and nurses who subjected them to "long judgmental and moralistic harangues on their habits and lifestyle." In fact, so many UC students consulted the Haight-Ashbury clinic that it earned the nickname Berkeley Annex. To gain the trust and confidence of young people, the Haight-Ashbury Free Clinic provided "informality of both décor and manner" and maintained the "strictest regard for the confidential character of personal records and problems. Patient-doctor relationships were relaxed, and the greatest possible use was made of hippie volunteers" from local colleges, schools, and the community. The staff also believed that clients needed to have as much input as possible in health care delivery and regularly consulted with former patients and other area young people to ensure that their needs were being met.[73]

The success of the Haight-Ashbury Free Clinic inspired the creation of similar facilities near other college and university campuses. In Cambridge, Brenner was convinced of the need for such alternatives for students after an experience earlier that year, when a student consulted him for help with a friend: the woman had had a septic abortion, but when she sought treatment at a local hospital, she had received a long, humiliating lecture from a nurse who said she "deserved what she got, living the way she did, sleeping around, getting pregnant, and having an abortion." Brenner and Coles consulted with their counterparts in San Francisco for guidance and in late 1967 received a sixty-nine thousand dollar grant from New York City's Field Foundation to start the Cambridgeport Free Clinic. Although the clinic was intended primarily to serve those who were too poor and/or too alienated from society to use traditional health care services, the founders also believed its clinic would be useful to students from Harvard, Radcliffe, MIT, and other local institutions "who, for one reason or another, are dissatisfied" with university health systems.[74] Other cities and college towns in the United States and Canada followed the examples of San Francisco and Boston, and by 1973, North America had 175 such facilities, and clinic directors and personnel had formed the National Free Clinic Council, an information center and lobbying organization.[75]

Student Advisory Committees and Consumer Rights

Students who remained on campus for medical care demanded a greater say in how their health centers were run and the services they offered. During the 1960s and 1970s, a number of student health services created student advisory committees to better understand and serve student needs. Among the pioneers in this regard was UC Berkeley, which in 1960 created the Student Health Service Committee (SHSC) as part of the student government, the Associated Students of the University of California. The SHSC initially served "to maintain rapport between University students and their health facilities" as well as to organize health-related volunteer activities such as blood drives, collecting medicines for clinics in the developing world, and recruiting students to work as gofers for patients in the infirmary. By the mid-1960s, the SHSC had become more militant, lobbying the health center to provide reproductive health care and holding information sessions on such controversial topics as student drug use. In 1971 the committee demanded the ouster of psychiatric service director Dr. Harvey Powelson, whom they accused of using an "authoritarian approach" with both patients and staff.[76]

Among the most outraged students were members of the Rolling Quads, a group of paraplegic students formed in 1970 to lobby for the rights of the disabled. The group was led by Ed Roberts, the first severely physically disabled student to attend Berkeley (although the university had been offering services to blind students since the early 1950s). Roberts had contracted polio as a child and was completely paralyzed from the neck down and dependent on a iron lung while asleep. In 1962, the dean of students, Arleigh Williams, contacted Bruyn, the school's director of health services, about the possibility of Roberts attending the university and about how to care for him given his severe physical limitations. Bruyn believed that the only option was to house Roberts in the infirmary, the only location able to accommodate his iron lung and where he could receive round-the-clock medical attention and nursing care. Six months later, Berkeley admitted John Hessler, and within a year the hospital had fifteen men residing in the Cowell Hospital Program for disabled students. Roberts graduated in 1968 and became a part-time assistant to the dean of students, in charge of the Cowell Hospital Program. In 1970, the students asked to meet with Bruyn in the ward, where Roberts announced, "Well, Dr. Bruyn, I want to tell you that we've organized and we're taking over." One reason for their rebellion was their treatment by the main rehabilitation counselor, Lucile Withington, who objected to their clothing, long hair, and visits by "undesirable" friends at all hours, disrupting her strict hospital routine. In addition, Powelson had ordered the eviction of those who were not following the program's rules—most notably, those prohibiting use of alcohol—and were failing to attend class and maintain minimum academic standards. When the students protested their eviction, Powelson threatened to have them committed to a psychiatric ward for observation. Like other student organizations at this time, the Rolling Quads took their protest to the streets of Berkeley, eventually prompting the university to create the Physically Disabled Students Program, the first "program for quads, run by quads."[77]

At the University of North Carolina, Chapel Hill, students created a Student Health Service Administrative Board in 1971 in response to horror stories about the health service. In 1975, the board published a Health Consumers Handbook aimed at setting minimal standards for the health service and giving students a more active role in ensuring that the university's health service met their needs: "These standards will give the consumer a basis for what to expect in certain circumstances, how to evaluate treatment and what to do if services do not comply with the standards."[78]

In 1970, the ACHA recognized the growing consumer power of students by establishing the Task Force on Students and College Health, funded by a ninety-eight thousand dollar grant from the U.S. Department of Health, Education, and Welfare. The task force consisted of students from various institutions in different parts of the country who were charged with developing a position paper that give insight into student health services "through the eyes of the consumer." The association also reserved two hundred places at the Fifth National Conference on College Health for student participants. Unlike previous conferences, these students would be bona fide representatives of their institutions' student advisory committees and were allowed to be full registrants who could participate in all aspects of the conference. The ACHA's president, Robert W. Gage, acknowledged that some of his colleagues claimed that students with no training in the health professions would be unable to offer "any useful advice concerning the delivery of medical care" but countered that "only the consumer can reflect and interpret accurately the rising expectations for health which are shared by the entire community. Access to a high-quality health program is being accepted rapidly as a fundamental right of all citizens," he declared, "not only those who are able to command adequate services in time of need." If students "are expected to pay the bill for the program," he argued, "they should have a major role in setting priorities and developing the specifics of services which are offered." Finally, students with a say in medical care would not only encourage "wise and timely use of services" but also "assist in developing and sustaining support, both private and public, for the comprehensive health programs which they have helped to formulate."[79] Cultivating public support for student health services was becoming more difficult, however, as a consequence of major economic and political shifts in the 1970s.

Backlash and Budget Cuts

In 1973, Baltimore psychiatrist Kent E. Robinson wrote, "There are many signs that health, counseling, and psychiatric services, as well as other student personnel services, are seriously threatened at scores of American colleges and universities." Budgetary problems and the escalating cost of medical care had forced the University of Wisconsin to close its entire counseling service and Texas Tech to shut down its infirmary; other colleges in the West were considering similar measures. The University of Missouri had disbanded its student health center as a separate entity and merged it with the medical school. In California, the budget for all counseling and medical services at public institutions of higher education had been slashed, a measure that led Bruyn to resign from the directorship of the Berkeley health service. The Michigan state legislature had passed a resolution stating that the state colleges and universities would only provide health care on a fee-for-service basis, which meant that institutions with minimal services could not expand them and that those with adequate services would have to retrench because students who lacked health insurance could not afford fee-for-service care. In Maryland, where Robinson served as a psychiatric consultant to several Baltimore-area colleges, several state college administrators considered a similar move, arguing that "colleges should not be in the business of providing health care that duplicates private health service." Robinson argued that such an attitude ignored the fact that even if a student could pay for medical care in the community, doing so meant taking valuable time away from classes and academic work. The end result of this policy, he argued, would be inadequate health care for most students. The reluctance of state legislatures to raise college budgets, Robinson observed, resulted at least in part "to continuing legislative ire over student demonstrations." Legislators, he wrote, were reluctant to fund services that would indulge and coddle "impudent" students. Yet budgetary concerns alone did not explain the "enthusiasm with which some college presidents have embraced proposals to dismantle all student services." Rather, the attack on in loco parentis by students had given administrators license to abolish all services "that have nothing to do with education." What troubled him most was the fact that "no one is giving any thoughtful consideration to separating the student personnel services that can logically be discontinued as outmoded from those which ought to continue in spite of financial pressures because of their supportive value."[80]

Students also continued to attack student health services, complaining about long waits, inconvenient hours, and lack of courtesy from harried staff.[81] Students were especially angry when health service fees skyrocketed to make up for reductions in state and federal funds. At Berkeley, students hoped their role in hiring one of their own as health service director—1969 graduate James Brown—would make the service more responsive to their needs. While Brown was the most progressive director up to that point—he even agreed to offer abortion services free of charge—students felt betrayed when budget cuts under Governor Ronald Reagan forced the health service to dramatically increase student health fees. After the cost of health care was raised by $150 a year in 1974, Andrew E. Wade wrote angrily to the *Daily Californian*, "As a student, I have the right to a justification for such a radical increase in the cost of a service, which, due to today's cost of medical aid, is a necessity of life." Added Wade, "When I questioned personnel at Cowell Hospital, they 'passed the buck' to Blue Cross."[82] At the University of North Carolina, Chapel Hill, student body president J. B. Kelly and Student Health Service Advisory Board member Kathleen Pointer wrote to the trustees in 1979 that the 53 percent increase in student health fees was "exorbitant" and came without any input from students. "Inflation is not a fantasy," Pointer wrote, and the increase violated wage and price controls set by the Carter administration and approved by the UNC Board of Trustees.[83]

Concerns about the rising costs of health care once again placed college health squarely in the middle of national debates about federally funded health care insurance. In 1972, the ACHA received an eighty-five hundred dollar grant from the Commonwealth Fund to study college health services as part of a larger assessment of the nation's health care system. According to Dr. Samuel I. Fuenning of the University of Nebraska, support from the fund allowed the ACHA to make "considerable progress" toward defining goals and standards that reflected those set by the Health Maintenance Act of 1973 and current debates over national health insurance. "In view of the recently enacted HMO legislation and pending probable national health insurance," Fuenning stated, "the Association is now directing its attention to the implications of these in respect to college health." Fuenning expressed hope that the study would have "some input into the thinking of Congressional staff members who are preparing or thinking about proposals for national health insurance." This would allow the organization to continue its efforts "to develop comprehensive health services, including maintenance and prevention services, for student health programs at colleges and universities around the country."[84]

At the same time, ACHA members wanted to ensure that the push for health care reform did not ignore the special concerns of college students. As ACHA executive director James Dilley declared at a 1976 conference on college health programs sponsored by the Josiah Macy Jr. Foundation, college and university health services had pioneered and continued to operate on the model of what was essentially a health maintenance organization (HMO). He was encouraged by the passage of the HMO Act of 1976, which symbolized that Congress had made this model a "matter of national policy." Yet he also expressed concern that the act's cost-containing measures would make it difficult for campus health services, which served over 9 million students, "to be nurtured and permitted to grow." Dilley encouraged his colleagues to "become more adroit in our justification of a health service delivery system that serves a unique segment of that society."[85]

The campaign for national health insurance in the 1970s was no more successful than similar movements earlier in the century, as various constituencies bickered over various health care plans.[86] Once again, college physicians were called on to change with the times. In his 1981 presidential address, "New Realities: The Challenge to Change," before the ACHA, Dr. H. Spencer Turner instructed his colleagues to find solutions to a number of significant changes in the student body: the growing number of nontraditional students; reduced financial support for higher education; new responsibilities involving environmental health and safety; and ongoing debates about national health care. Although he emphasized the great progress made over the previous century, he also noted that a "glaring omission" in discussions of national health care in the early 1980s was the "over 11 million men and women who use college health services as their primary source of medical care." On the contrary, it was "painfully obvious" that "national healthcare planners have, in no realistic way, considered this large group that constitutes nearly 5% of the population." He concluded, "If we are to make the point of the need for our continued existence at institutions of higher education, we must again indicate to administrators, to organized medicine . . . that we do have a role to play and that we are viable."[87] It would not be long before a new plague would surface to underscore once again the relevance of college health services.

CHAPTER 8

College Health since the 1980s: The Lessons of History

In 1995, Dr. Richard P. Keeling, director of University Health Services at the University of Wisconsin in Madison, observed that the AIDS epidemic had put the ACHA "on the map." Dealing with this health crisis over the previous decade had brought college health services into closer contact with other student affairs personnel but also had exposed the "limits of rules and regulations." In addition, the epidemic brought to the surface prejudices about homosexuality, forcing health professionals to reexamine their assumptions as well as reiterate policies and procedures regarding confidentiality. Although strategies for dealing with HIV provoked public outcry, college health centers "discovered that we could manage—and survive—controversy." Most importantly, the search for solutions to the AIDS crisis allowed college health professionals to become "less isolated" as they created new networks and task forces for dealing with the epidemic.[1]

As with the earlier social hygiene campaign of the 1920s, college health professionals had to confront broader cultural prejudices about diseased "others"—in this case, the "4-H Club" of homosexuals, heroin users, hemophiliacs, and Haitians, among whom the disease first surfaced in the United States. According to Keeling, the fact that the disease appeared primarily among groups often ostracized by mainstream society ensured that an "epidemic of fear" would accompany the medical epidemic.[2] In 1985, recognizing that college health services needed to take the lead in stemming panic over AIDS, the ACHA created the Task Force on AIDS to provide recommendations and guidelines for institutions formulating campus AIDS policies. That December, the ACHA released *General Statements on Institutional Response to AIDS*, in which the organization attempted to set guidelines for institutional policies. Believing that the main response to the epidemic should be education, the task force hoped to give students, faculty, and administrators accurate information about AIDS and its transmission and thereby to dispel popular misconceptions that the disease could be caught through casual contact in the classroom or dormitory. The ACHA also insisted that students with AIDS or those who tested positive for HIV had the same rights to privacy as did other medical cases.[3]

Unlike the earlier social hygiene campaign, however, students played a prominent role in developing AIDS policies on college campuses, part of the legacy of student demands for reproductive health services in the 1960s and 1970s. Following the example set by other student groups, gay and lesbian organizations staged sit-ins and other protests against institutional discrimination. In 1971, the National Student Association continued its tradition of supporting politically sensitive issues, passing its first gay rights mandate at the group's twenty-fourth National Student Congress.[4] Two years later, years of pressure from gay rights organizations such as the Student Homophile League at Columbia led the trustees of the American Psychiatric Association to finally remove homosexuality from the *Diagnostic and Statistical Manual*. By the mid-1980s, gay and lesbian students had gained a certain level of respect and recognition from both their peers and administrators. Although discrimination and homophobia continued, the days of denying admission to or expelling homosexual students were over. Some gay and lesbian activists even gained places in student government. Randy Shilts, who would later gain fame for his exposé on the early years of the AIDS epidemic, was an openly gay member of the student government at the University of Oregon who fought successfully for greater recognition of the rights of homosexual students on campus.[5]

Among the first student-run AIDS education projects was the one started by the Gay and Lesbian Alliance at Stanford, one of the country's oldest gay student groups. The group's approach to AIDS awareness emulated the irreverence of student-initiated self-help efforts during the 1960s and 1970s, promoting a "sex positive" approach to disease prevention. The director of the Stanford AIDS Education Project, Jeff Zinman hoped that by "eroticizing safe sex," the project's programs would change behavior as well as extend AIDS education beyond the homosexual community. "The thing about safe sex is that it's good for anyone who's sexually active with many partners," Zinman explained. "Safe sex won't get you pregnant. Safe sex won't transmit any sexually transmitted disease. It's not just about AIDS."[6]

At the University of California, Berkeley, the student health service started an AIDS education program in the spring of 1985 in response to calls from students concerned that they might be HIV positive as well as to reports of discrimination against gay and lesbian students and faculty, who were perceived to be at higher risk for the disease. The health service soon enlisted the help of campus student activists to develop an AIDS prevention guide, thereby providing leadership in the campus's response to the crisis. In an "Open Letter to the University and College Community" that served as the guide's preface, student editor Terry Weisser declared, "When we strip away the myths about AIDS, one truth remains clear: AIDS can be prevented." To stop the spread of the disease, he argued, campuses had to provide information about disease prevention in a "nonjudgmental manner." Echoing earlier public health campaigns regarding college students' central role in promoting awareness and shaping public opinion, Weisser wrote that although students comprised only 5 percent of the total population, they constituted a "vital resource" that could influence public opinion outside the academy.[7]

Within a few years, AIDS education programs had become so ubiquitous that one student interviewed in 1993 quipped, "Most of my generation knew about AIDS before they were sexually active. It's always been there for us. You know, the "sex = death" generation? That's us."[8] Because the infection rate among heterosexuals in the United States and Western Europe remained extremely low (0.2 percent), fears that the disease would spread into the general population gradually disappeared. For the few infected American students, the development of antiretroviral drugs turned AIDS into a manageable, chronic illness rather than the virtual death sentence it was in the 1980s and early 1990s. Consequently, AIDS once again became a disease of the "other," occurring in other countries, in other cultures, and among those who engage in sexual practices and lifestyles other than the white, Western, heterosexual "norm."[9]

Although the impact of AIDS on the general population fell short of expectations, it did have some effect on sexual practices. Studies of condom usage showed an increase from 12 percent in 1975 to nearly 50 percent in 1989 among college students, compared with only 8 percent growth during that time period among the general population. Fears of infection with human papilloma virus (HPV), the most common sexually transmitted disease, led to intensified disease prevention programs, including recommendations that all women aged between eleven and twenty-six be vaccinated against HPV. Other sexually transmitted diseases—such as chlamydia, gonorrhea, and genital herpes—also remained prevalent. Researchers found that a myth of "personal invulnerability" as well as "safe sex fatigue" reduced students' willingness to follow medical advice regarding disease prevention. Male students seemed especially doctor averse, leading some experts in college health to call once again for initiatives to reduce the gender gap in college health services by creating men's clinics and implementing other strategies to induce male students to seek health care.[10]

At the same time, college health experts identified another epidemic: the growing mental health crisis on college campuses. With the passage of the Americans with Disabilities Act (1990) and the development of new psychotropic prescription medications, college health programs found themselves dealing with significant numbers of students with chronic mental illness who previously would not have been able to attend college.[11] A study conducted by the counseling service at Kansas State University found that between 1988 and 2001, the number of students with documented depression doubled and the proportion of students taking psychiatric medication rose from 10 to 25 percent.[12] The ACHA's National College Health Assessment issued in spring 2006, which surveyed ninety-five thousand students on 117 campuses, found that 16 percent of the students reported depression so severe they found it difficult to function. Over 9 percent had seriously considered suicide, and one in every hundred had attempted suicide in the previous year.[13]

Lawsuits brought by families of students who had committed suicide created additional challenges for college mental health services. The Family Educational Rights and Privacy Act and the Health Insurance Portability and Accountability Act prevented mental health services from releasing medical records without the student's consent. Students at George Washington University and Hunter College filed lawsuits under state and federal antidiscrimination law after being barred from campus following suicide attempts. Both institutions settled out of court and were compelled to change their policies regarding mandatory leaves for suicidal students. In March 2007, Virginia became the first state in the nation to pass legislation prohibiting colleges and universities from expelling or punishing students "solely for attempting to commit suicide, or seeking mental-health treatment for suicidal thoughts or behaviors." The horrifying murder-suicide at Virginia Tech the following month, which caused the deaths of thirty-two students and faculty plus the gunman, intensified the dilemma of how to identify and treat at-risk students without violating students' privacy rights or federal disability law. Mental health experts argued that the best way to prevent future tragedies was to reduce the stigma associated with mental illness and reassure students that they would not be punished for seeking counseling services.[14]

ACHA members used these health risks faced by modern students to justify the continued viability of college health programs. During the campaign for national health insurance during the early 1990s, college health experts once again explicitly linked the national crisis over access to health care and the college population. "College students are among the most poorly insured groups in America," wrote Kevin Patrick, director of student health services at the University of California at San Diego, "with from 20 to 30 percent without *any* medical coverage." Furthermore, college students no longer represented an elite portion of the population but came from a variety of ethnic and socioeconomic groups. Poor health and lack of access to adequate medical care created a significant barrier to regular college attendance. The escalating cost of health care merely exacerbated the situation, thus creating an "unconscionable circumstance" where many young people lacked access to even the most basic health services.[15]

These financial concerns led some institutions to divest themselves altogether from the health care business. Complaining about the cost and "distraction" of running campus health centers, some institutions of higher education outsourced student health care to health maintenance organizations and other external health care providers.[16] At the same time, wealthy institutions continued to recognize that comprehensive health services were a powerful marketing tool, especially for a new generation of "helicopter parents." Student affairs personnel found that even those who had protested in loco parentis in their own youth were insisting on a more active role in the daily lives of their children, especially if the parents were footing the bill.[17]

These recent trends illustrate continuities with the past as well as how far the field of college health has come in terms of addressing the needs of a heterogeneous student body. This book has shown that at its best, the evolution of college health has been part of a larger historical process of bringing "outsiders in." As historian Paula Fass forcefully argues, the history of American education "is crucially related to the problems associated with American diversity." Therefore, to understand fully the history of education in our society, we must thoroughly examine the history of how outsiders gained access to educational institutions.[18]

This book has argued that the body is another locus through which reformers have attempted to open higher education to outsiders. The earliest college health programs emerged to address concerns about the impact of higher education on the female body. The Civil War and later

World War I and World War II directed similar attention to the integrity of male bodies, thereby justifying similar hygiene programs for college men. The centrality of physical and mental health to educational aspirations was reinforced by *Higher Education for American Democracy: The Report of the President's Commission on Higher Education* (1947), which called for a massive expansion of higher education to promote American ideals of democracy and equality of opportunity. In addition to recommending an end to racial and religious discrimination, increases in financial aid programs, and creation of community colleges, the report stated that promotion of physical and mental health constituted a central part of the mission of higher education. Today's college health and student affairs professionals continue to reiterate this relationship between health services and equality of access to higher education. Some observers have argued that health services not only help the individual student but can improve an institution's bottom line by enhancing student retention.[19]

Yet much has changed since the early twentieth century, when college health programs were justified as being integral to a college or university's role as a surrogate for the parental home. College health experts continue to argue that their services need to be developmentally appropriate and that the purpose of college health programs—as well as of higher education more generally—is to foster a "bridge toward independence."[20] Defining what is "developmentally appropriate" for college students is tricky. Older students do not fall within the Society for Adolescent Medicine's definition of a college freshman as a "high school senior without parents around."[21] In fact, a significant percentage of students are parents themselves.

This book has shown that health programs in higher education have met with the most success when they allow students to have input on health initiatives rather imposing them from the top down. This notion of direct student involvement is a fairly recent development, since the original argument in favor of campus health services was that they were part of an institution's responsibility in loco parentis. During the 1960s, this model became unacceptable to a generation of students rebelling against paternalism both in institutions of higher education and in American society more generally. Many campus health centers responded to these student protests by creating student health advisory committees. The ACHA created a student task force and later a student section as vehicles for student participation in the organization. These efforts to recruit students as advocates for campus health services continue today, as illustrated by a recent issue of *Student Health Spectrum* emphasizing students' role in student health.[22]

Finally, college health programs continue to play a vital role in the broader community. Since the early twentieth century, college health professionals have sided with larger social movements for universal access to the benefits of modern medicine. Like other progressives in medicine and public health, those in college health have argued that medical care is a right, not a privilege. This view has brought college health into broader initiatives for universal health care. Although the emphasis on protecting the minds and bodies of America's best and brightest has at times been elitist, the larger message that students educated in the principles of modern medicine and hygiene would go on to demand a higher standard of public health in their own homes and communities was for its day quite progressive. This historic link between college health and the public health is exemplified today by the Association of American Colleges and Universities Program for Health and Higher Education, which seeks not only to reduce the incidence of HIV, drug and alcohol use, smoking, and health problems affecting the college population but also to help students become "active and effective civic and moral agents, exercising their responsibilities in the world of work, in the civic arena, and in their personal lives."[23]

Maintaining and reaffirming this connection between "inside" and "outside" is important because many of the most common health issues faced by modern students—obesity, smoking, diabetes, lack of exercise, respiratory illnesses—are no different than those affecting the adult population as a whole. Other issues—most notably alcohol use and sexually transmitted diseases—are products of complex sociocultural factors both on and off campus. For most students, the college experience is not limited to a discrete life stage of semidependency between adolescence and adulthood. Repeated cycles of economic boom and bust combined with the demand for a highly trained workforce to compete in a global marketplace means that growing numbers of students drift in and out of institutions of higher education, leaving and returning as finances and family responsibilities allow. These "nontraditional" students are also more likely to have heavy work and family responsibilities and thus face additional physical and mental stress while having less time for exercise and other health-promoting behaviors. Again, these problems are not unique to college students, yet as in the past, college health programs can serve as models for the larger culture. Thus, college health today not only can help to bring outsiders in by ensuring a health status compatible with academic success but also can bring the inside of the academy out to the larger world by using college health services as a model for improving public health for the nation as a whole.

Notes

CHAPTER 1

1. Caille Millner, "Young Women Hear Mixed Signals at Harvard and Beyond," Pacific News Service, 21 January 2005, available online at http://www.imdiversity.com/villages/woman/careers_workplace_employment/pns_summers_wo men_0105.asp, accessed 20 June 2006.

2. Linda Kerber, *Women of the Republic: Intellect and Ideology in Revolutionary America* (Chapel Hill: University of North Carolina Press, 1986), 199–200.

3. Joan Jacobs Brumberg, *Mission for Life* (New York: Free Press, 1980), 20, 79–80.

4. Quoted in Thomas Woody, *A History of Women's Education in the United States.* (New York: Science, 1929), 2:99.

5. Helen Lefkowitz Horowitz, *Alma Mater: Design and Experience in the Women's Colleges from Their Beginnings to the 1930s* (Boston: Beacon, 1984), 23–24.

6. Edward H. Clarke, *Sex in Education; or, A Fair Chance for the Girls* (Boston: Osgood, 1873). For more on the impact of Clarke's ideas on female higher education, see Sheila Rothman, *Woman's Proper Place: A History of Changing Practices, 1870 to the Present* (New York: Basic Books, 1978); Rosalind Rosenberg, *Beyond Separate Spheres: Intellectual Roots of Modern Feminism* (New Haven: Yale University Press, 1982); Carroll Smith-Rosenberg, *Disorderly Conduct: Visions of Gender in Victorian America* (New York: Knopf, 1985); Cynthia Eagle Russett, *Sexual Science: The Victorian Construction of Womanhood* (Cambridge: Harvard University Press, 1989); Sue Zschoche, "Dr. Clarke Revisited: Science, True Womanhood, and Female Collegiate Education," *History of Education Quarterly* 29, no. 4 (1989): 545–69.

7. Mary Putnam Jacobi, *The Question of Rest for Women during Menstruation* (New York: Putnam's, 1877), 227.

8. For more on Jacobi's life and work, see Carla Jean Bittel, "The Science of Women's Rights: The Medical and Political Worlds of Mary Putnam Jacobi" (Ph.D. diss., Cornell University, 2003).

9. Barbara Gutman Rosencrantz, *Public Health and the State: Changing Views in Massachusetts* (Cambridge: Harvard University Press, 1972), 71.

10. Nathan Allen, *The Education of Girls, as Connected with Their Growth and Development* (Boston: Bicknell, 1879), 34–35.

11. Ibid., 35.

12. Harvey Green, *Fit for America: Health, Fitness, Sport, and American Society* (New York: Pantheon, 1986); James C. Whorton, *Crusaders for Fitness: The History of American Health Reformers* (Princeton: Princeton University Press, 1982); Martha Verbrugge, *Able-Bodied Womanhood: Personal Health and Social Change in Nineteenth-Century Boston* (New York: Oxford University Press, 1988); Joan Burbick, *Healing the Republic: The Language of Health and the Culture of Nationalism in Nineteenth-Century America* (New York: Cambridge University Press, 1994).

13. Quoted in Horowitz, *Alma Mater*, 29. See also Debra Herman. "College and After: The Vassar Experiment in Women's Education, 1861–1924" (Ph.D. diss., Stanford University, 1979).

14. Edward H. Clarke, *Sex in Education*, 79–85.

15. For more on the relationship between physiological research and physical education at this time, see Roberta Park, "Physiologists, Physicians, and Physical Educators: Nineteenth Century Biology and Exercise, *Hygienic* and *Educative*," *Journal of Sport History* 14, no. 1 (1987): 28–60.

16. Quoted in Woody, *History of Women's Education*, 2:118.

17. Barbara Sicherman, "The Paradox of Prudence: Mental Health in the Gilded Age," *Journal of American History* 62, no. 4 (1976): 890–912.

18. Alida C. Avery to Edward H. Clarke, 4 November 1873, in *Sex and Education: A Reply to Dr. E. H. Clarke's "Sex in Education,"* ed. Julia Ward Howe (Boston: Roberts, 1874), 191–95.

19. Alida C. Avery, "Vassar College," in *Education of American Girls, Considered in a Series of Essays*, ed. Anna C. Brackett (New York: Putnam, 1874), 356.

20. Quoted in Herman, "College and After," 10–11.

21. M. Carey Thomas, "Present Tendencies in Women's College and University Education," *Educational Review* 25 (January 1908): 68.

22. Alice Freeman Palmer, "Three Types of Women's Colleges," in George Herbert Palmer and Alice Freeman Palmer, *The Teacher: Essays and Addresses on Education* (Boston: Houghton Mifflin, 1908), 324–25.

23. S. T. Rorer, "What College Girls Eat," *Ladies Home Journal*, November 1908, 13.

24. Horowitz, *Alma Mater*, 82–94, 105–16.

25. Society for the Collegiate Instruction of Women, *Secretary's Annual Report, Fourteenth Year* (1892–93), 9.

26. S. Weir Mitchell, "Address to Radcliffe Students," 17 January 1895, Class of 1899 Collections, Alumnae Association, RG IX, ser. 7, Radcliffe College Archives, Schlesinger Library, Institute for Advanced Study, Cambridge, Massachusetts.

27. Radcliffe College Annual Report, 1893, 13, Schlesinger Library, Radcliffe Institute for Advanced Study, Cambridge, Massachusetts.

28. Horowitz, *Alma Mater*, 237–47.

29. James Allen Young, "Height, Weight, and Health: Anthropometric Study

of Human Growth in Nineteenth-Century American Medicine," *Bulletin of the History of Medicine* 53, no. 2 (1979): 214–16.

30. Sophie M. Hartley, "The Influence of Higher Education upon Women with Reference to Their Ability to Propagate Healthy Species," *Woman's Medical Journal* 4, no. (1895): 319–21; Mary Roberts Smith, "Statistics of College and Non-College Women," *Publications of the American Statistical Association* 7, no. 49–50 (1900): 1–26; Mabel Newcomer, "Physical Development of Vassar College Students, 1884–1920," *Publications of the American Statistical Association* 17, no. 136 (1919–20): 976–82.

31. Dudley Allen Sargent, "The Relation of Physical Education to Race Betterment," in *Proceedings of the First National Conference on Race Betterment* (Battle Creek, Mich.: Gage, 1914), 104–6. See also Dudley Allen Sargent, "The Physical Development of Women," *Scribner's*, February 1889, 172–85.

32. Dudley Allen Sargent, *Dudley Allen Sargent: An Autobiography*, ed. Ledyard W. Sargent (Philadelphia: Lea and Febiger, 1927), 148.

33. Verbrugge, *Able-Bodied Womanhood*, 133–35.

34. Albert Shaw, "Physical Culture at Wellesley," *American Review of Reviews* 6 (1892): 549. See also C. H. Cook, "The Effect of College Life at Wellesley," *Medical Communications of the Massachusetts Medical Society* 16 (1893): 191–95.

35. Anna J. MacKeag, "Methods in Use in Colleges for Women for the Maintenance and Advancement of the Health of Students," *Woman's Medical Journal* 23, no. 9 (1913): 199. See also Clara Gregory Baer, "Health of College Women," in *Proceedings of the National Education Association of the United States* (1916), 690–93; Annie O'Hagan, "The Athletic Girl," *Munsey's*, August 1901, 729–38; Edith Rickert, "Has the College Injured the Health of Girls?" *Ladies' Home Journal*, January 1912, 11–12.

36. Sophia F. Richardson, "Tendencies in Athletics for Women in Colleges and Universities," *Popular Science Monthly*, February 1897, 517–26.

37. Anna G. Howes, *Health Statistics of Women College Graduates: Report of a Special Committee of the Association of Collegiate Alumnae* (Boston: Wright and Potter, 1885).

38. Quoted in Mary O. Nutting, "Mount Holyoke," in *Education of American Girls*, ed. Brackett, 324.

39. G. Stanley Hall, *Adolescence: Its Psychology and Its Relation to Physiology, Anthropology, Sociology, Sex, Crime, Religion, and Education* (New York: Appleton, 1904), 2:631, 637.

40. Jurgen Herbst, *And Sadly Teach: Teacher Education and Professionalization in American Culture* (Madison: University of Wisconsin Press, 1989).

41. Barbara Miller Solomon, *In the Company of Educated Women: A History of Women in Higher Education* (New Haven: Yale University Press, 1985), 46–54.

42. Charlotte Conable, *Women at Cornell: The Myth of Equal Education* (Ithaca: Cornell University Press, 1977), 72, 81, 101–2.

43. Helen Lefkowitz Horowitz, *Campus Life: Undergraduate Cultures from the End of the Eighteenth Century to the Present* (Chicago: University of Chicago Press, 1987), 201.

44. Lynn D. Gordon, *Gender and Higher Education in the Progressive Era* (New Haven: Yale University Press, 1990), 94–99.

45. Martin Meyerson and Dilys Pegler Winegrad, *Gladly Learn and Gladly Teach: Franklin and His Heirs at the University of Pennsylvania, 1740–1976* (Philadelphia: University of Pennsylvania Press, 1978), 124, 213.

46. Solomon, *In the Company of Educated Women*, 43–61.

47. Rebecca S. Montgomery, *The Politics of Education in the New South: Women and Reform in Georgia* (Baton Rouge: Louisiana State University Press, 2006).

48. Richard Meckel, "Going to School, Getting Sick: The Social and Medical Construction of School Diseases in the Late Nineteenth Century," in *Formative Years: Children's Health in the United States, 1880–2000*, ed. Alexandra Minna Stern and Howard Markel (Ann Arbor: University of Michigan Press, 2002), 186. See also John Duffy, "Mental Strain and Overpressure in the Schools: A Nineteenth-Century Viewpoint," *Journal of the History of Medicine and Allied Sciences* 23, no. 1 (1968): 63–79; John Duffy, "School Buildings and the Health of American School Children in the Nineteenth Century," in *Healing and History: Essays for George Rosen*, ed. Charles Rosenberg (New York: Science History, 1979): 161–78.

49. Charles Nutt, *History of Worcester and Its People*, vol. 4 (New York: Lewis Historical, 1919), available online at http://www.rootsweb.com/~maworces/wohistbk/nutt4.htm, accessed 29 March 2005.

50. Mary J. Studley, *What Our Girls Ought to Know* (New York: Holbrook, 1878), 10.

51. Regina Markell Morantz-Sanchez, *Sympathy and Science: Women Physicians in American Medicine* (New York: Oxford University Press, 1985); Toby Appel, "Physiology in American Women's Colleges: The Rise and Decline of a Female Subculture," *Isis* 85, no. 1 (1994): 26–56; Ellen Singer More, *Restoring the Balance: Women Physicians and the Profession of Medicine* (Cambridge: Harvard University Press, 1999).

52. Geraldine Jonçich Clifford, ed., *Lone Voyagers: Academic Women in Coeducational Universities, 1870–1937* (New York: Feminist, 1989), 12.

53. Jana Nidiffer, *Pioneering Deans of Women: More Than Wise and Pious Matrons* (New York: Teachers College Press, 2000), 2, 56–57.

54. Elizabeth Griego, "The Making of a 'Misfit': Clelia Duel Mosher, 1863–1940," in *Lone Voyagers*, ed. Clifford, 147–82.

55. Clelia Duel Mosher, "The Schematogram—A New Method of Graphically Recording Posture and Changes in the Contours of the Body," *School and Society* 1 (1915): 642–45.

56. Clelia Duel Mosher, "The Height of College Women," *Medical Woman's Journal* 28 (November 1921): 274–76. See also Clelia Duel Mosher, "The Muscular Strength of College Women," *Journal of the American Medical Association* 70, no. 3 (1918): 140–42; Clelia Duel Mosher, "Some of the Causal Factors in the Increased Height of College Women," *Journal of the American Medical Association* 81 (1923): 535–38.

57. Clelia Duel Mosher, "The Physical Training of Women in Relation to Functional Periodicity," *Woman's Medical Journal* 25, no. 4 (1915): 3–5, 9, 11; Clelia Duel Mosher, "A Physiologic Treatment of Congestive Dysmenorrhea and Kindred Disorders Associated with Menstrual Function," *Journal of the American Medical Association* 62 (1914), 1297–1301.

58. Note, 18 November 1927, Clelia Duel Mosher Papers, box 1, folder 4, Stanford University Special Collections, Stanford, California.

59. Jane Snyder to Clelia Duel Mosher, 16 June 1929, Mosher Papers, box 1, folder 6.

60. Clelia Duel Mosher, *Woman's Physical Freedom* (New York: Woman's Press, 1923), 84–87; Clelia Duel Mosher, *Health and the Woman Movement* (New York: Young Women's Christian Associations, 1916).

61. Mary Roberts Smith to Carnegie Institution, 20 September 1905, Mosher Papers, box 2, folder 1.

62. Havelock Ellis to Clelia Duel Mosher, 25 September 1901, Mosher Papers, box 1, folder 6.

63. G. Stanley Hall to Clelia Duel Mosher, 2 October 1905, Mosher Papers, box 2, folder 1.

64. Dorothy Gies McGuigan, *A Dangerous Experiment: 100 Years of Women at the University of Michigan* (Ann Arbor: University of Michigan, 1970), 11, 33–36.

65. Lynn D. Gordon, *Gender and Higher Education*, 52–65.

66. Mary Bennett Ritter, *More Than Gold in California, 1849–1933* (Berkeley, Calif.: Professional, 1933), 201–17.

67. Robert Samuel Fletcher, *A History of Oberlin College from Its Foundation through the Civil War* (Oberlin, Ohio: Oberlin College, 1943); Carol Lasser, ed., *Educating Men and Women Together: Coeducation in a Changing World* (Urbana: University of Illinois Press, 1987).

68. Henry N. Drewry, *Stand and Prosper: Black Colleges and Their Students* (Princeton: Princeton University Press, 2001).

69. Glenda Gilmore, *Gender and Jim Crow: Women and the Politics of White Supremacy in North Carolina, 1896–1920* (Chapel Hill: University of North Carolina Press, 1996), 40–41.

70. Margaret A. Lowe, *Looking Good: College Women and Body Image, 1875–1930* (Baltimore: Johns Hopkins University Press, 2003), 13–15.

CHAPTER 2

1. Quoted in Nathan Allen, *Physical Culture in Amherst College* (Lowell, Mass.: Stone and Huse, 1869), 4–5.

2. Benjamin Franklin, *Proposals Relating to the Education of Youth in Pennsylvania* (Philadelphia, 1749).

3. Frederick Rudolph, *The American College and University: A History* (New York: Knopf, 1962), 24–27.

4. Edward M. Hartwell, *Physical Training in American Colleges and Universities* (Washington, D.C.: U.S. Government Printing Office, 1885), 15–23.

5. Edward Hitchcock Jr. to Burges Johnson, 6 December 1906, Edward (AC 1849) and Mary Judson Hitchcock Family Papers, ser. 4, subser. A, Incoming Correspondence, box 14, folder 28, Amherst College Archives and Special Collections, Amherst, Massachusetts.

6. Allen, *Physical Culture in Amherst College*, 10.

7. "President Eliot on Amherst College," *Harvard Register*, March 1880, 61.

8. Claude Moore Fuess, *Amherst: The Story of a New England College* (Boston: Little, Brown, 1935).

9. Edward Hitchcock Sr., *An Essay on Alcoholic and Narcotic Substances, as Articles of Common Use, Addressed Particularly to Students* (Amherst, Mass.: Adams, 1830).

10. Quoted in Stephen Nissenbaum, *Sex, Diet, and Debility in Jacksonian America* (Westport, Conn.: Greenwood, 1980), 44.

11. For more on the growth of the sex trade and concerns about young male sexual behavior at this time, see Patricia Cline Cohen, *The Murder of Helen Jewett* (New York: Vintage, 1998). For more on concerns about masturbation, see Ben Barker-Benfield, "The Spermatic Economy: A Nineteenth-Century View of Sexuality," *Feminist Studies* 1, no. 1 (1972): 45–74; Charles E. Rosenberg, "Sexuality, Class, and Role in Nineteenth-Century America," *American Quarterly* 25, no. 2 (1973): 131–53; John S. Haller and Robin M. Haller, *The Physician and Sexuality in Victorian America* (New York: Norton, 1974),196; Tristam H. Engelhardt, "The Disease of Masturbation: Values and the Concept of Disease," *Bulletin of the History of Medicine* 48, no. 2 (1974): 234–38; R. P. Neuman, "Masturbation, Madness, and the Modern Concepts of Childhood and Adolescence," *Journal of Social History* 8, no. 3 (1976): 1–27; Gail Pat Parsons, "Equal Treatment for All: American Medical Remedies for Male Sexual Problems, 1850–1900," *Journal of the History of Medicine and Allied Sciences* 32, no. 1 (1977): 55–71; Robert Darby, "The Masturbation Taboo and the Rise of Routine Male Circumcision: A Review of the Historiography," *Journal of Social History* 36, no. 3 (2003): 737–57.

12. Quoted in Nissenbaum, *Sex, Diet, and Debility*, 44.

13. Nicolaas A. Rupke, *Richard Owen: Victorian Naturalist* (New Haven: Yale University Press, 1994).

14. John Harley Warner, "Ideals of Science and Their Discontents in Late Nineteenth-Century American Medicine," *Isis* 82, no. 313 (1991): 460.

15. Edward Hitchcock Jr., *A Report of Twenty Years Experience in the Department of Physical Education at Amherst College* (Amherst, Mass.: Bangs, 1881), 5–7.

16. Report to the Trustees for 1864–65, Papers Connected with the Department of Physical Education at Amherst College, vol. 1, Amherst College Archives and Special Collections, Amherst, Massachusetts (hereafter cited as DPEAC).

17. Tony Ladd and James A. Mathisen, *Muscular Christianity: Evangelical Protestants and the Development of American Sport* (Grand Rapids, Mich.: Baker, 1999), 14, 38.

18. Report of the Department of Physical Education of 1865–66 to the Trustees, DPEAC, vol. 1.

19. Edward Hitchcock Jr. to Nathan Allen, 10 September 1868, DPEAC, vol. 1.

20. Quoted in Hitchcock, *Physical Culture in Amherst College*, 20.

21. Edward Hitchcock Jr., "Hygiene at Amherst College," *American Public Health Association Papers and Reports* 4 (1877–78): 50–55.

22. Levi H. Elwell to Edward Hitchcock Jr., 5 July 1910, Hitchcock Papers, ser. 4, subser. A, Incoming Correspondence, box 10, folder 11.

23. Edward Hitchcock Jr. to Nathan Allen, 10 September 1868, DPEAC, vol. 1.

24. Nathan Allen to Edward Hitchcock Jr., 20 January 1862, Hitchcock Papers, ser. 4, subser. A, Incoming Correspondence, box 10, folder 3.

25. James Allen Young, "Height, Weight, and Health," 219.

26. Nathan Allen, *Changes in New England Population* (Lowell, Mass.: Stone, Huse, 1877). For more on Allen's impact on population studies, see William Leach, *True Love and Perfect Union: The Feminist Reform of Sex and Science* (New York: Basic Books, 1980), 329.

27. James Allen Young, "Height, Weight, and Health," 223.

28. First Report of the Professor of Physical Education and Hygiene to the Corporation of Amherst College, 5 July 1862, DPEAC, vol. 1.

29. Hitchcock, *Report of Twenty Years Experience,* 12.

30. John F. Kazan, *Houdini, Tarzan, and the Perfect Man: The White Male Body and the Challenge of Modernity in America* (New York: Hill and Wang, 2001), 10–13.

31. Sargent, *Dudley Allen Sargent,* 17.

32. Ibid., 61–62.

33. Ibid., 100–101, 131.

34. Ibid., 143–46.

35. Ibid., 148, 156.

36. Ibid., 165.

37. Ibid., 196, 207–8.

38. Robert W. Rydell, *All the World's a Fair: Visions of Empire at American International Expositions, 1876–1916* (Chicago: University of Chicago Press, 1984), 57; Jacqueline Urla and Alan C. Swedlund, "The Anthropometry of Barbie: Unsettling Ideals of the Feminine Body in Popular Culture," in *Deviant Bodies: Critical Perspectives on Difference in Science and Popular Culture,* ed. Jennifer Terry and Jacqueline Urla (Bloomington: Indiana University Press, 1995), 288–89.

39. R. Tait McKenzie, "The Search for Physical Perfection," in *University Lectures Delivered by Members of the Faculty in the Free Public Lecture Course, 1914–1915* (Philadelphia: University of Pennsylvania, 1915), 409–19.

40. R. Tait McKenzie, *Exercise in Education and Medicine* (Philadelphia: Saunders, 1909), 132.

41. Ibid., 174.

42. R. Tait McKenzie, "Physical Education at the University of Pennsylvania—from 1904 to 1931—and the Gates Plan," *Research Quarterly* 3, no. 1 (1932): 19–20.

43. Ibid., 20–21.

44. Larry Owens, "Pure and Sound Government: Laboratories, Playing Fields, and Gymnasia in the Nineteenth-Century Search for Order," *Isis* 76, no. 2 (1985):182–94.

45. Roberta J. Park, "Research Note: Edward M. Hartwell and Physical Training at the Johns Hopkins University, 1879–1890," *Journal of Sport History* 14, no. 1 (1987): 108–19.

46. Hartwell, *Physical Training,* 9, 152–53.

47. The term *body project* comes from Joan Jacobs Brumberg, *The Body Project: An Intimate History of American Girls* (New York: Vintage, 1998).

48. Kazan, *Houdini, Tarzan, and the Perfect Man,* 4–6.

49. For example, see James C. Whorton, "'Athlete's Heart': The Medical Debate over Athleticism," *Journal of Sport History* 9, no. 1 (1982): 30–52.

50. McKenzie, *Exercise in Education and Medicine*, 181–82.

51. Martin Summers, *Manliness and Its Discontents: The Black Middle Class and the Transformation of Masculinity, 1900–1930* (Chapel Hill: University of North Carolina Press, 2004), 243–52.

52. Horowitz, *Campus Life*, 25–27.

53. "Dr. Mitchell on Athletics: Address before the New York City Alumni Association, 16 January 1906," S. Weir Mitchell Papers, MSS 2/0241–03, ser. 7, box 16, FF 7.2, College of Physicians of Philadelphia Historical Library, Philadelphia.

54. President's Annual Report, Harvard College, 1878–79, 65, Harvard University Archives, Cambridge, Massachusetts.

55. Horowitz, *Campus Life*, 23–55.

56. Nidiffer, *Pioneering Deans of Women*, 65–66.

57. Hitchcock, "Hygiene at Amherst College," 51.

58. Edward Hitchcock Jr., "The Department of Physical Education and Hygiene in Amherst College," *Massachusetts State Board of Health Reports* 10 (1879): 72.

59. Hitchcock, "Hygiene at Amherst College," 52–53.

60. Hitchcock, "The Department of Physical Education," 72.

CHAPTER 3

1. George A. Soper, "The Epidemic of Typhoid Fever at Ithaca, N.Y.," *Journal of the New England Water Works Association* 18, no. 4 (1905): 431–33.

2. Nancy Tomes, *The Gospel of Germs: Men, Women, and the Microbe in American Life* (Cambridge: Harvard University Press, 1998), 30.

3. Rosencrantz, *Public Health and the State*, 70.

4. Judith Walzer Leavitt, *Typhoid Mary: Captive to the Public Health* (Boston: Beacon, 1996).

5. Samuel Hopkins Adams, "Typhoid: An Unnecessary Evil," *McClure's*, June 1905, 145, 150–52.

6. Tomes, *Gospel of Germs*, 30.

7. Morris Bishop, *A History of Cornell* (Ithaca: Cornell University Press, 1962), 78, 293.

8. Ibid., 334, 442–43.

9. "A Lesson from the Fire," *Cornell Daily Sun*, 10 December 1906, 4.

10. Nidiffer, *Pioneering Deans of Women*, 66.

11. Mrs. E. Dennett to Jacob Gould Schurman, n.d., Typhoid Fever Epidemic (Ithaca, NY) Records, 1901–1906, Cornell University, Division of Rare Books and Manuscripts, Ithaca, New York (hereafter cited as Typhoid Records).

12. Quoted in Michael P. McCarthy, *Typhoid and the Politics of Public Health in Nineteenth-Century Philadelphia* (Philadelphia: American Philosophical Society, 1987), 3.

13. Edward Potts Cheyney, *History of the University of Pennsylvania, 1740–1940* (Philadelphia: University of Pennsylvania Press, 1940), 395.

14. Meyerson and Winegrad, *Gladly Learn and Gladly Teach*, 204, 213.

15. University of Pennsylvania, *The Dormitory System as Designed by Cope and Stewardson, Architects* (Philadelphia: privately printed, 1895), 4–5.

16. Ibid., 224.

17. Ibid., 6–7.

18. Cheyney, *History of the University of Pennsylvania*, 340.

19. E. Digby Baltzell, *Philadelphia Gentlemen: The Making of a National Upper Class* (New Brunswick, N.J.: Transaction, 1989); Richard Angelo, "The Students at the University of Pennsylvania and the Temple College of Philadelphia, 1873–1906: Some Notes on Schooling, Class, and Social Mobility in the Late Nineteenth Century," *History of Education Quarterly* 19, no. 2 (1979): 179–205.

20. Edwin E. Slosson, *Great American Universities* (New York: Macmillan, 1910), 362.

21. Alex Duke, *Importing Oxbridge: English Residential Colleges and American Universities* (New Haven: Yale University Press, 1996), 50–51.

22. Cheyney, *History of the University of Pennsylvania*, 340–44.

23. Duke, *Importing Oxbridge*, 52.

24. This concept of an agrarian myth comes from Rudolph, *American College and University*, 95–96.

25. Carol U. Sisler, Margaret Hobbie, and Jane Marsh Dieckmann, eds., *Ithaca's Neighborhoods: The Rhine, the Hill, and the Goose Pasture* (Ithaca, N.Y.: Dewitt Historical Society of Tompkins County, 1988), 9; Henry Edward Abt, *Ithaca* (Ithaca, N.Y.: Kellogg, 1926), 148. Population grew from 5,628 in 1865 to more than 13,000 in 1903.

26. For more on Silent City, see Carol Kammen, *The Peopling of Tompkins County: A Social History* (Interlaken, N.Y.: Heart of the Lakes, 1985), 165, 193–95.

27. Sisler, Hobbie, and Dieckmann, *Ithaca's Neighborhoods*, 8.

28. Soper, "Epidemic," 434–35.

29. "Pollution of the City's Water," *Ithaca Daily Journal*, 2 March 1903, 3.

30. Luzerne Coville, "Ithaca Epidemic of 1903," *American Medicine*, 9 January 1904, 67; Mervin T. Sudler, "The Recent Epidemic of Typhoid Fever in Ithaca, New York," *Philadelphia Medical Journal*, 11 April 1903, 632. Reports on the condition of the city water are included in the Minutes of the Board of Health, 1901, 1902, Ithaca City Hall, Ithaca, New York.

31. For further discussion of the antimonopoly sentiments during this time, see Robert H. Wiebe, *The Search for Order, 1877–1920* (New York: Hill and Wang, 1967); Richard Hofstader, *The Age of Reform* (New York: Knopf, 1955).

32. Dorothy Harris, *History of Ithaca's Water and Sewer Systems* (Ithaca, N.Y.: Department of Public Works, Water and Sewer Division, 1956), 2–4; Abt, *Ithaca*, 135–36; Nathan Matthews and Mynderse Van Cleef, *The City of Ithaca v. Ithaca Water Works Co., et. al.: Brief for the Defendants* (Boston: Ellis, 1906), 6–9.

33. Tomes, *Gospel of Germs*, 48–66.

34. Soper, "Epidemic," 444.

35. Ibid.

36. Bishop, *History of Cornell*, 203–5.

37. David Schiller, "The Social History of the 1903 Typhoid Epidemic: A

Study in Anger and Action," unpublished paper, 1973, 13–14, Cornell University Archives, Ithaca, New York.

38. V. A. Moore and Emile Chamot to Jacob Gould Schurman, 19 February 1903, G. S. Williams to Jacob Gould Schurman, 19 February 1903, Typhoid Records.

39. *Ithaca Daily News*, 26 January 1903, 4; *Ithaca Daily News*, 6 February 1903, 4; *Cornell Alumni News*, 4 February 1903, 140; Soper, "Epidemic," 433; Coville, "Ithaca Epidemic," 67.

40. *Cornell Alumni News*, 25 February 1903, 59, 62.

41. Report of the Trustees of Cornell University, 21 April 1903, Typhoid Records.

42. Soper, "Epidemic," 440.

43. For references to "gangs of laborers," see, for example, *Ithaca Daily News*, 4 February 1903, 1; *Ithaca Daily News*, 11 February 1903, 3; *Ithaca Daily News*, 13 February 1903, 4; *Ithaca Daily News*, 10 April 1903, 6. For accounts of the "filthy habits" of the immigrant workers, see Elias J. Durand, H. H. Whetzel, and H. M. Van Hook to V. A. Moore, n.d., Typhoid Records.

44. Accusations of links between Cornell and the water company appeared almost daily. See, for example, *Ithaca Daily News*, 7 February 1903, 1; *Ithaca Daily News*, 19 February 1903, 4; *Ithaca Daily News*, 7 March 1903, 5; *Ithaca Daily News*, 9 March 1903, 5; *Ithaca Daily News*, 11 March 1903, 4; *Ithaca Daily News*, 17 March 1903, 4; *Ithaca Daily News*, 19 March 1903, 4.

45. "Blame for Ithaca Epidemic," *New York Times*, 27 February 1903, 8.

46. Schurman speech, 19 February 1903, in *Cornell Daily Sun*, 20 February 1903, 1.

47. Andrew Carnegie to Jacob Gould Schurman, 13 March 1903, Typhoid Records.

48. *Cornell Alumni News*, 15 April 1903, 213.

49. Arturo Bravo to Jacob Gould Schurman, 14 May 1903, Typhoid Papers; "Carnegie Fund for Students: One Draft Presented Which Was Not Paid," *Ithaca Journal*, 21 May 1903.

50. *Cornell Daily Sun*, 18 February 1903, 2; *Cornell Alumni News*, 18 February 1903, 152.

51. Schurman speech, 19 February 1903, in *Cornell Daily Sun*, 20 February 1903, 1.

52. Jacob Gould Schurman to parents, 24 February 1903, Typhoid Records.

53. *Ithaca Daily News*, 3 March 1903, 5.

54. Mrs. W. U. Bateman to Jacob Gould Schurman, 24 July 1903, Typhoid Records.

55. Edward L. Prime to Jacob Gould Schurman, 16 February 1906, Typhoid Records.

56. Viviana Zelizer, *Pricing the Priceless Child: The Changing Social Value of Children* (New York: Basic Books, 1985), 134–35.

57. Bishop, *History of Cornell*, 405.

58. *Cornell Alumni News*, 25 March 1903, 191; *Cornell Alumni News*, 22 April 1903, 220; Bishop, *History of Cornell*, 359–61.

59. Conable, *Women at Cornell*, 110–11.

60. Jennifer L. Gunn, "Factory Work for Doctors: The Early Years of the Section on Industrial Medicine and Public Health of the College of Physicians of Philadelphia," *Transactions and Studies of the College of Physicians of Philadelphia* 17 (1995): 61–93; Angela Nugent, "Fit for Work: The Introduction of Physical Examinations in Industry," *Bulletin of the History of Medicine* 57, no. 4 (1983): 578–95; Amy Fairchild, *Science at the Borders: Immigrant Medical Inspection and the Shaping of the Modern Industrial Labor Force* (Baltimore: Johns Hopkins University Press, 2003).

61. President's Annual Report, Harvard College, 1877–78, 25, Harvard University Archives, Cambridge, Massachusetts.

62. Annah May Soule, "Relation of the School and College to Health," *School Review* 11 (1903): 817–26.

63. David O. Levine, *The American College and the Culture of Aspiration, 1915–1940* (Ithaca: Cornell University Press, 1986), 135–61.

64. Warren E. Forsythe, "Health Service in American Colleges and Universities," *Journal of the American Medical Association* 63, no. 22 (1914): 1928.

65. Gail Bederman, *Manliness and Civilization: A Cultural History of Gender and Race in the United States, 1880–1917* (Chicago: University of Chicago Press, 1995).

66. Fairchild, *Science at the Borders*, 7.

67. Thomas A. Storey, *The Status of Hygiene Programs in Institutions of Higher Education in the United States* (Stanford, Calif.: Stanford University Press, 1927), 50–69.

68. President's Annual Report, Harvard College, 1893–94, 38–39, Harvard University Archives, Cambridge, Massachusetts.

69. G. F. Reinhardt, "University of California Infirmary Student Health Protection," in *Fourth International Congress on School Hygiene*, ed. Thomas A. Storey, Frederic Allen Woll, and Julian Park (Buffalo, N.Y.: Courier, 1914), 161.

70. First Report of the Professor of Physical Education and Hygiene to the Corporation of Amherst College, 5 July 1862, DPEAC, vol. 1.

71. "Hygiene at Amherst College: Experience of the Department of Physical Education and Hygiene in Amherst College for the Past 16 Years," Hitchcock Papers, box OSB5, folder 10.

72. George Rosen, "Contract or Lodge Practice and Its Influence on Medical Attitudes to Health Insurance," *American Journal of Public Health* 67, no. 4 (1977): 374–78; Gunn, "Factory Work for Doctors."

73. Robert T. Legge, "Students' Health Insurance at the University of California," in *Proceedings of the Conference on Social Insurance, Called by the International Association of Industrial Accident Boards and Commissions* (Washington, D.C.: U.S. Government Printing Office, 1917), 505.

74. Warren E. Forsythe, "Student Health Work," *School and Society* 4 (1916): 439.

75. *Cornell Alumni News*, 25 February 1903, 59, 62.

76. Ruth Boynton, "Historical Development of College Health Services," *Student Medicine* 10 (1962): 294–305.

77. Joseph E. Raycroft, "Safeguarding the Health of College Students," *Science*, n.s. 39, no. 1011 (1914): 709.

78. Rosemary Stevens, *In Sickness and in Wealth: American Hospitals in the Twen-*

tieth Century (Baltimore: Johns Hopkins University Press, 1989), 138.

79. John Sundwall, "Organization and Activities of a University Health Service," *School and Society* 4 (1916): 348–49.

80. Beatrix Hoffman, *The Wages of Sickness: The Politics of Health Insurance in Progressive America* (Chapel Hill: University of North Carolina Press, 2001), 9.

81. Orrin Leslie Elliott, *Stanford University: The First Twenty-five Years* (Stanford, Calif.: Stanford University Press, 1937), 216–19; Students' Guild Records, Stanford University Special Collections, Stanford, California.

82. Forsythe, "Health Service," 1927.

83. University Board of Health to Benjamin Ide Wheeler, 10 February 1902, Office of the President, University Board of Health Records, ser. 1, box 13, folder 3, Bancroft Library, University of California, Berkeley.

84. George F. Reinhardt to Warren Olney, 20 July 1911, Board of Regents Records, CU-1, box 88, folder 23, Bancroft Library, University of California, Berkeley.

85. "Prytanean Society," *Daily Californian*, 26 August 1901, 3.

86. *The Prytaneans: An Oral History of the Prytanean Society and Its Members and Their University, 1901–1920* (Berkeley, Calif.: Prytanean Alumnae, 1970), 27.

87. Ritter, *More Than Gold in California*, 215–17.

88. George F. Reinhardt to Benjamin Ide Wheeler, 24 February 1905, Board of Regents Records, CU-1, box 69, folder 9, Bancroft Library, University of California, Berkeley.

89. "Hospital Plans Are Changed," *Daily Californian*, 18 February 1902, 1; *Daily Californian*, 18 February 1902, 2.

90. *Prytaneans*, 27.

91. Legge, "Students' Health Insurance at the University of California," in *Proceedings*, 505. See also Robert T. Legge, "Students' Health Insurance at the University of California," *California State Journal of Medicine* 15, no. 4 (1917): 102–4; Edith Shatto King, "Health Insurance in a Student Community," *Survey* 36 (1916): 619–20.

92. "Regents Establish University Hospital," *Daily Californian*, 20 August 1906, 1. For more on the earthquake's impact on the university, see Janet Ruyle, "The 1906 Earthquake and Its Aftermath in Berkeley," *Chronicle of the University of California*, no. 1 (1998): 24–48.

93. J. Arthur Myers, *Masters of Medicine: An Historical Sketch of the College of Medical Sciences, University of Minnesota, 1888–1966* (St. Louis: Green, 1968), 592.

94. Susan L. Smith, *Sick and Tired of Being Sick and Tired: Black Women's Health Activism in America, 1890–1950* (Philadelphia: University of Pennsylvania Press, 1995), 18.

CHAPTER 4

1. "Editorial: School and College Contracts," *American Medical Association Bulletin*, June 1927, 1.

2. Robyn Muncy, *Creating a Female Dominion in American Reform, 1890–1935* (New York: Oxford University Press, 1991); Rothman, *Woman's Proper Place*.

3. H. E. Robertson, "Problems Confronting the Organization of a University

Public Health Service," in *Fourth International Conference on School Hygiene*, ed. Storey, Woll, and Park 140.

4. John Sundwall, "The Interrelationship between Physical Education and Students' Health Service," *American Physical Education Review*, 1921, 172–79.

5. William A. Christmas and John M. Dorman, "The Storey of College Health Hygiene: Thomas A. Storey, MD (1875–1943) and the Promotion of Hygiene," *Journal of American College Health* 45, no. 1 (1996): 31.

6. Warren E. Forsythe, *Health Service in American Colleges and Universities* (Ann Arbor: University of Michigan, 1926), 12–14.

7. Tomes, *Gospel of Germs*, 237–45.

8. Boynton, "Historical Development of College Health Services."

9. Executive Committee of the New York Women's Committee, Princeton Endowment Fund, "Why Princeton Needs a New Infirmary," n.d., Historical Subject Files, Box 279/F: McCosh Infirmary General, 1916–1990, Seeley G. Mudd Manuscript Library, Princeton University, Princeton, New Jersey, available online at http://www.med.umich.edu/medschool/chm/influenza/assets/pdfs/princeton/mudd01.pdf, accessed 6 March 2007.

10. "John Sundwall, 1880–1950, Memorial Assembly, April 19, 1951," John Sundwall Papers, box 1, Bentley Historical Library, University of Michigan, Ann Arbor.

11. Myers, *Masters of Medicine*, 592.

12. University of Minnesota Board of Regents Minutes, 15 March 1918, courtesy of Paul Rupprecht, director, Boynton Health Service, University of Minnesota.

13. Tim Brady, "The Great Flu Epidemic," *Minnesota Magazine*, January–February 2005, available online at http://www.alumni.umn.edu/3Jan20057.html, accessed 26 July 2005.

14. Myers, *Masters of Medicine*, 594.

15. Marion LeRoy Burton to John Sundwall, 28 May 1921, Sundwall Papers, box 1.

16. John Sundwall, "The Teaching of College Hygiene," *American Journal of Public Health* 17, no. 1 (1927): 48–49.

17. A. D. Browne to John Sundwall, 19 January, 18 February 1922, Sundwall Papers, box 1.

18. William H. Geer to John Sundwall, 21 December 1921, Sundwall Papers, box 1.

19. John Sundwall to John B. Grant, 1 November 1921, Sundwall Papers, box 1.

20. Eugene C. Howe, "The Health of the College," *American Journal of Public Health* 9 (1919): 755.

21. Harold S. Diehl, "Research Opportunities in Student Health Work," in *Proceedings of the American Student Health Association*, 1927, 69–70, American College Health Association Library, Linthicum, Maryland.

22. John Sundwall to D. F. Smiley, 22 December 1932, Sundwall Papers, box 4.

23. R. W. Bradshaw, "Research in Student Health," *American Journal of Public Health* 19 (1929): 1229.

24. Steven J. Peitzman, "Why Support a Women's Medical College? Philadelphia's Early Male Medical Pro-Feminists," *Bulletin of the History of Medicine* 77, no. 3 (2003): 576–99.

25. "John Sundwall, 1880–1950, Memorial Assembly, April 19, 1951," Sundwall Papers, box 1.

26. Sarah Parker White to Marion Hague Rea, 2 March 1933, American Student Health Association Papers, Stanford University, Special Collections, box 5, folder 4 (hereafter cited as ACHA Records).

27. Marjorie Wagoner to D. F. Smiley, 12 January 1929, ACHA Records, box 6, folder 11.

28. Estelle Freedman, "Separatism as Strategy: Female Institution Building and American Feminism, 1870–1930," *Feminist Studies* 5, no. 3 (1979): 512–29; Morantz-Sanchez, *Sympathy and Science;* Rosenberg, *Beyond Separate Spheres;* Margaret W. Rossiter, *Women Scientists in America: Struggles and Strategies to 1940* (Baltimore: Johns Hopkins University Press, 1982).

29. Marion Hague Rea to D. F. Smiley, 21 January 1929, ACHA Records, box 6, folder 11.

30. Marjorie Jeffries Wagoner to Warren E. Forsythe, 11 March 1930, ACHA Records, box 6, folder 10.

31. William P. Shepard, "Ruth Evelyn Boynton, M.D.," *Journal-Lancet* 84 (1964): 355–56.

32. Nidiffer, *Pioneering Deans of Women,* 107–23.

33. Ibid., 79.

34. Leslie A. Loveless, "A Fraternity for Women," *Minnesota Medicine,* September 2003, available online at http://www.mmaonline.net/publications/MNMed2003/September/Loveless.html, accessed 26 July 2005.

35. William P. Shepard, "Ruth Evelyn Boynton," 357.

36. Harold S. Diehl to L. D. Coffman, 9 July 1935, University Health Service Records, AD5.1, folder 5, University Archives, Andersen Library, University of Minnesota, Minneapolis.

37. William P. Shepard, "Ruth Evelyn Boynton," 355–58.

38. Morantz-Sanchez, *Sympathy and Science.*

39. Kathy Robbins, Julia Ann Kelly, and Edward Ehlinger, "Pioneer in Student Health Services," *Minnesota Medicine,* September 2003, available online at www.mnmed.org/publications/MNMed2003/September/Robbins.html, accessed 9 April 2007.

40. Judson Knight, "Paul Bertau Cornely," in *Notable Black American Scientists* (Detroit: Gale, 1999), 80–83; Paul B. Cornely, interview, 1977, Paul Bertau Cornely Papers, accession #2001-133, box 2, National Library of Medicine, Bethesda, Maryland.

41. Forsythe and Cornely collaborated on an unpublished study, "An Analysis of Hygiene Administration and Education at the University of Michigan," 1937, University Health Service Records, box 2, Bentley Historical Library, University of Michigan, Ann Arbor.

42. Karen Anderson, "Brickbats and Roses: Lucy Diggs Slowe, 1883–1937," in *Lone Voyagers,* ed. Clifford, 284.

43. Dorothy Boulding Ferebee, interview by Merze Tate, 28, 31 December

1979, in *The Black Women Oral History Project* (Cambridge, Mass.: Schlesinger Library, Radcliffe College, 1984), 457–58.

44. Ibid., 472.

45. Patricia Bell-Scott, "To Keep My Self-Respect: Dean Lucy Diggs Slowe's 1927 Memorandum on the Sexual Harassment of Black Women," *National Women's Studies Association Journal* 9, no. 2 (1997): 70–77.

46. Anderson, "Brickbats and Roses," 290.

47. Rayford W. Logan, *Howard University: The First Hundred Years, 1867–1967* (New York: New York University Press, 1969), 336.

48. Ferebee, interview by Tate, 472.

49. Ibid., 458.

50. William P. Shepard, "Ruth Evelyn Boynton," 357.

51. Ferebee, interview by Tate, 472–73.

52. Knight, "Paul Bertau Cornely," 80–83.

53. Ruth Boynton to O. F. Hedley, 29 November 1937, ACHA Records, box 7, folder 2.

54. Henry H. Moore to John Sundwall, 22 May 1926, Sundwall Papers, box 1.

55. Henry H. Moore to John Sundwall, 15 November 1927, Sundwall Papers, box 1. For more on the CCMC, see I. S. Falk, "Medical Care in the USA—1932–1972," *Milbank Memorial Fund Quarterly* 51, no. 1 (1973): 1–39; Milton I. Roemer, "I. S. Falk, the Committee on the Costs of Medical Care, and the Drive for National Health Insurance," *American Journal of Public Health* 75, no. 8 (1985): 841–48; Forrest A. Walker, "Americanism versus Sovietism: A Study of the Reaction to the Committee on the Costs of Medical Care," *Bulletin of the History of Medicine* 53, no. 4 (1979): 489–504.

56. I. S. Falk to John Sundwall, 11 July 1931, Isidore S. Falk Papers, ser. II, box 31, folder 38, Manuscripts and Archives Division, Sterling Library, Yale University, New Haven, Connecticut.

57. I. S. Falk to John Sundwall, 28 November 1930, Sundwall Papers, box 4.

58. Don M. Griswold and Hazel I. Spicer, *University Student Health Services* (Publications of the Committee on the Costs of Medical Care 19; Chicago: University of Chicago Press, 1932), 108, 110.

59. Report of Executive Committee to CCMC, 18 December 1931, Falk Papers, ser. II, box 32, folder 57.

60. Olin West to John Sundwall, 1 December 1932, Sundwall Papers, box 4.

61. G. Stanley Hall, "Student Customs," *Proceedings of the American Antiquarian Society* n.s. 14 (1900): 105.

62. Seneca Egbert, "Medical Service in Colleges and Universities," in *Proceedings of the American Student Health Association*, 1927, 35, American College Health Association Library, Linthicum, Maryland.

63. Paul C. Phillips, "Care of Students' Health at Amherst College," in *Fourth International Congress on School Hygiene*, ed. Storey, Woll, and Park, 5:133, 139.

64. Charles E. Rosenberg, *The Care of Strangers: The Rise of America's Hospital System* (New York: Basic Books, 1987).

65. John Sundwall to Edwin Fauver, 23 January 1922, Sundwall Papers, box 1.

66. Fred N. Miller, "Off to College," *Hygeia* 5 (1927): 500–502; D. F. Smiley, "The Health of Your Boy in College," Hygeia 4 (1926): 554–58; Earl F. Morris,

"Going to College for Your Health," *Hygeia* 8 (1930): 801–4; Calvin T. Ryan, "If I Were Selecting a College," *Hygeia* 12 (1934): 778–80; Thomas D. Wood, "How Much Do College Graduates Know about Health?" *Hygeia* 2 (1924): 113–14; J. Rosslyn Earp, "Hygiene in an American College," *Hygeia* 2 (1924): 613–14; "Illness as Cause of College Failures," *Hygeia* 4 (1926): 413; Marie B. Ryan, "A College Training in Health," *Hygeia* 4 (1926): 575–78; "Plain Facts about Health and Disease," *Hygeia* 6 (1928): 406–7; Harold S. Diehl, "Health Exams for College Students," *Hygeia* 8 (1930): 51–54; Rose Henderson, "Colleges and Health," *Hygeia* 11 (1933): 777–79.

67. Harry G. Robinson and Hazel Ruth Edwards, *The Long Walk: The Placemaking Legacy of Howard University* (Washington, D.C.: Moorland-Spingarn Research Center, Howard University, 1996), available online at http://www.howard.edu/longwalk, accessed 9 April 2007.

68. Paul B. Cornely, "The Status of Student Health Programs in Negro Colleges in 1938–39," *Journal of Negro Education* 10, no. 2 (1941): 155.

69. Isolation Hospital Log Books, Rauner Special Collections Library, Dartmouth College, Hanover, New Hampshire.

70. Quoted in Theodor Swanson, *The Story of Dick's House* (Lunenburg, Vt.: Stinehour, 1977), 13, 15, 17.

71. Ferebee, interview by Tate, 457–58.

72. Boynton, "Historical Development of College Health Services," 296.

73. American Medical Association, Bureau of Medical Economics, *University and College Health Centers* (Chicago: American Medical Association, 1936), 17.

CHAPTER 5

1. *Report of the United States Interdepartmental Social Hygiene Board for Fiscal Year Ended June 30, 1920* (Washington, D.C.: U.S. Government Printing Office, 1921), 84–85.

2. Thomas A. Storey, "The Work of the United States Interdepartmental Social Hygiene Board," *Social Hygiene* 5, no. 4 (1919): 441–60; Thomas A. Storey, "A Summary of the United States Interdepartmental Social Hygiene Board," *Social Hygiene* 7, no. 1 (1921): 59–76.

3. Muncy, *Creating a Female Dominion;* Rothman, *Woman's Proper Place.*

4. Nancy Bristow, *Making Men Moral: Social Engineering during the Great War* (New York: New York University Press, 1996), 187–89.

5. Thomas A. Storey, *The Status of Hygiene Programs in Institutions of Higher Education in the United States* (Stanford, Calif.: Stanford University Press, 1927) The quotations are from pp. 11–12. For biographical information on Storey, see Christmas and Dorman, "Storey of College Health Hygiene."

6. The term *cultural authority* comes from Paul Starr, *The Social Transformation of American Medicine* (New York: Basic Books, 1982), 13–15.

7. Sundwall, "Teaching of College Hygiene," 49.

8. Paula S. Fass, *The Damned and the Beautiful: American Youth in the 1920s* (New York: Basic Books, 1977); Beth Bailey, *From Front Porch to Back Seat: Courtship in Twentieth-Century America* (Baltimore: Johns Hopkins University

Press, 1988); Vern Bullough, *Science in the Bedroom: A History of Sex Research* (New York: Basic Books, 1994), 112–21.

9. Clelia Duel Mosher, *The Mosher Survey: Sexual Attitudes of Forty-five Victorian Women* (New York: Arno, 1980). Mosher described similar changes among Stanford coeds in her diary (Mosher Papers, SC 11, box 1, folder 10). See also Katherine Bement Davis, *Factors in the Sex Life of Twenty-two Hundred Women* (New York: Harper, 1929).

10. Summers, *Manliness and Its Discontents*, 272, 244, 276.

11. Christina Simmons, "African Americans and Sexual Victorianism in the Social Hygiene Movement, 1910–1940," *Journal of the History of Sexuality* 4 (1993): 51–75.

12. Jeffrey P. Moran, *Teaching Sex: The Shaping of Adolescence in the Twentieth Century* (Cambridge: Harvard University Press, 2000), 23–32.

13. Storey, *Status of Hygiene Programs*, 7.

14. Charles W. Eliot, "The American Social Hygiene Association," *Journal of Social Hygiene* 1, no. 1 (1914): 3.

15. G. Stanley Hall, "Education and the Social Hygiene Movement," *Journal of Social Hygiene* 1, no. 1 (1914): 30.

16. G. Stanley Hall, "The Teaching of Sex in Schools and Colleges," *Social Diseases* 2, no. 4 (1911): 1–19.

17. Quoted in Moran, *Teaching Sex*, 74–75.

18. David P. Setran, "Student Religious Life in the 'Era of Secularization': The Intercollegiate YMCA, 1877–1940," *History of Higher Education Annual* 21 (2001): 7–45.

19. Jodi Vandenberg-Daves, "The Manly Pursuit of a Partnership between the Sexes: The Debate over YMCA Programs for Women and Girls, 1914–1933," *Journal of American History* 78, no. 4 (1992): 1324–46; John Donald Gustav-Wrathall, *Take the Young Stranger by the Hand: Same-Sex Relations and the YWCA* (Chicago: University of Chicago Press, 1998).

20. Max J. Exner, "Program and Policy for Sex Education in the Colleges and Universities," typescript, 1915, Offices of Mssrs. Rockefeller, RG 2, ser. R, box 24, folder 250, Rockefeller Archive Center, North Tarrytown, New York (hereafter cited as OMR).

21. Max J. Exner to John D. Rockefeller, 18 October 1912, OMR, box 21, folder 210.

22. Max J. Exner, "Sex Education by the Young Men's Christian Association in Universities and Colleges," *Journal of Social Hygiene* 1, no. 4 (1915): 573. For more on the YMCA and sex education for younger children and adolescents, see Alexandra M. Lord, "Models of Masculinity: Sex Education, the United States Public Health Service, and the YMCA, 1919–1924," *Journal of the History of Medicine and Allied Sciences* 58, no. 2 (2003) 123–52; Alexandra M. Lord, "Naturally Clean and Wholesome: Women, Sex Education, and the United States Public Health Service, 1918–1928," *Social History of Medicine* 17, no. 3 (2004): 423–41.

23. Charles Hurrey to John D. Rockefeller, 30 January 1913, OMR, box 21, folder 210.

24. Max J. Exner to John D. Rockefeller, 27 October 1914, OMR, box 21, folder 211.

25. Summers, *Manliness and Its Discontents*, 272, 244, 276.

26. Setran, "Student Religious Life," 11.

27. John D. Rockefeller to Max J. Exner, 29 December 1916, OMR, box 39, folder 426.

28. Katherine Bement Davis to John D. Rockefeller, 8 January 1918, OMR, box 39, folder 426.

29. "Social Dissipation in College," *Nation*, 16 July 1908, 47; Charles F. Thwing, "College Disorders—Their Cause and Cure," *Harper's Weekly*, 31 October 1908, 23.

30. Max J. Exner, "The College and Social Hygiene Education," in *Proceedings of the American Student Health Association*, 1925, 23–30, American College Health Association Library, Linthicum, Maryland.

31. Storey, *Status of Hygiene Programs*, 3–5.

32. American Social Hygiene Association, 23 February 1933, Bureau of Social Hygiene, ser. 3, subser. 2, Social Hygiene, box 7, folder 164, Rockefeller Archive Center, North Tarrytown, New York.

33. Quoted in Moran, *Teaching Sex*, 101.

34. "Muensterberg Vigorously Denounces Red Light Drama," *New York Times*, 14 September 1913, SM4.

35. Clelia Duel Mosher diary, 6 June 1926, Mosher Papers, SC 11, box 1, folder 10.

36. Today, the eugenics movement is considered a fringe science associated with the genocidal policies of Nazi Germany, but in the first forty years of the twentieth century, individuals from across the political spectrum in countries around the world adopted various eugenic ideas. Proponents ranged from the most conservative and bigoted members of the established white Protestant elite to such diverse radical thinkers as Emma Goldman, Helen Keller, Margaret Sanger, Charlotte Perkins Gilman, and W. E. B. Du Bois. These constituencies shared a belief that the scientific management of human reproduction could lead to the improvement of society as a whole. They differed markedly in how human propagation should be controlled. Some stressed negative eugenics in the form of confinement and sterilization of the insane, the feebleminded, and other "unfit" individuals. Others stressed positive eugenic measures, including improvements in public health and preventive medicine, to ensure that fit individuals from even the most deprived of circumstances would survive. The groundbreaking work on this point is Daniel Kevles, *In the Name of Eugenics: Eugenics and the Uses of Human Heredity* (New York: Knopf, 1985). Recent work in the history of eugenics has confirmed Kevles's point that the movement included not only those who supported the most extreme measures of race improvement, such as sterilization and euthanasia, but also those who promoted Progressive Era social reforms affecting public health. See Diane Paul, *Controlling Human Heredity: 1865 to the Present* (Atlantic Highlands, N.J.: Humanities Press, 1995); Edward J. Larson, *Sex, Race, and Science: Eugenics in the Deep South* (Baltimore: Johns Hopkins University Press, 1995); Ian Robert Digginbotham, *Keeping America Sane: Psychiatry and Eugenics in the United States and Canada, 1880–1940* (Ithaca: Cornell University Press, 1997); Leila Zenderland, *Measuring Minds: Henry Herbert Goddard and the Origins of American Intelligence Tests* (New York: Cambridge University Press, 1998); Wendy Kline, *Build-*

ing a Better Race: Gender, Sexuality, and Eugenics from the Turn of the Century to the Baby Boom (Berkeley: University of California Press, 2001); Alexandra Minna Stern, *Eugenic Nation: Faults and Frontiers of Better Breeding in Modern America* (Berkeley: University of California Press, 2005).

37. Louis I. Dublin, "The Significance of the Declining Birth Rate," *Science*, 1 March 1918, 201–10.

38. For more on eugenics programs at state land-grant institutions, see Barbara A. Kimmelman, "The American Breeders' Association: Genetics and Eugenics in an Agricultural Context, 1903–13," *Social Studies of Science* 13, no. 2 (1983): 163–204; Alan I. Marcus, "The South's Native Foreigners: Hookworm as a Factor in Southern Distinctiveness," in *Disease and Distinctiveness in the American South*, ed. Todd L. Savitt and James Harvey Young (Knoxville: University of Tennessee Press, 1988), 79–99; Marilyn Holt, *Linoleum, Better Babies, and the Modern Farm Woman, 1890–1930* (Albuquerque: University of New Mexico Press, 1995). For information on eugenics in college courses, see Hamilton Cravens, *The Triumph of Evolution: American Scientists and the Heredity-Environment Controversy, 1900–1941* (Philadelphia: University of Pennsylvania Press, 1978), 53; Steven Selden, "Education Policy and Biological Science: Genetics, Eugenics, and the College Textbook, c. 1908–1931," *Teachers College Record* 87, no. 1 (1985): 35–51.

39. Thomas A. Storey, "The Colleges Look at Hygiene," *Journal of Social Hygiene* 17, no. 7 (1931): 383.

40. Sargent, "Relation of Physical Education to Race Betterment," 106. See also Gordon T. Bowles, *New Types of Old Americans at Harvard and at Eastern Women's Colleges* (Cambridge: Harvard University Press, 1932); Clelia Duel Mosher, "Concerning the Size of Women: Preliminary Note with Special Reference to Height," *California State Journal of Medicine* 19 (1921): 53–54; Faith Fairfield Gordon, "Physical Measurements of One Thousand Smith College Students," *American Journal of Public Health* 20, no. 9 (1930): 963–68.

41. Carolyn Geisel, "The Race Betterment Movement in Women's Colleges," in *Proceedings of the First National Conference on Race Betterment*, 345–46.

42. Sundwall, "Teaching of College Hygiene," 48–50. See also John Sundwall, "What Physical Education Should Contribute to Race Betterment," in *Proceedings of the Third Race Betterment Conference* (Battle Creek, Mich.: Race Betterment Foundation, 1928), 704–14.

43. Marcus, "South's Native Foreigners," 83.

44. John Ettling, *The Germ of Laziness: Rockefeller Philanthropy and Public Health in the New South* (Cambridge: Harvard University Press, 1981), 146.

45. W. Reece Berryhill to M. J. Rosenau, 11 December 1936, Student Health Service Records, box 6, University Archives, Wilson Library, University of North Carolina at Chapel Hill.

46. Daylanne K. English, *Unnatural Selections: Eugenics in American Modernism and the Harlem Renaissance* (Chapel Hill: University of North Carolina Press, 2004), 48.

47. Louis I. Dublin, "Historical Development of the Birth Control Movement and Its Effect on the Birth Rate," typescript, ca. 1918, 18, Louis I. Dublin Papers, box 5, National Library of Medicine, Bethesda, Maryland.

48. Michelle Mitchell, *Righteous Propagation: African Americans and the Politics of*

Racial Destiny after Reconstruction (Chapel Hill: University of North Carolina Press, 2004), 103–4.

49. Thomas J. Ward, *Black Physicians in the Jim Crow South* (Fayetteville: University of Arkansas Press, 2003), 249.

50. "Program of Work with Negro Voluntary Agencies," December 1943, American Social Hygiene Association Papers, box 117, folder 7, Social Welfare History Archives, Anderson Library, University of Minnesota, Minneapolis (hereafter cited as ASHA Papers).

51. Walter Clarke, "Statement on the American Social Hygiene Association: Dr. Clarke's Remarks at the Opening of the Conference on Negro Health Problems," 22 November 1943, ASHA Papers, box 117, folder 5.

52. Edward H. Beardsley, *A History of Neglect: Health Care for Blacks and Mill Workers in the Twentieth-Century South* (Knoxville: University of Tennessee Press, 1987), 94.

53. Paul B. Cornely, "Health Education—An Urgent Need in Negro Colleges," *National Negro Health Newsletter* 8, no. 2 (1940): 11–14.

54. Susan Smith, *Sick and Tired of Being Sick and Tired,* 149–51.

55. Ferebee, interview by Tate, 457.

56. Quoted in August Meier and Elliott Rudwick, *Black History and the Historical Profession* (Urbana: University of Illinois Press, 1986), 49. For a similar reading of the "transformation" of the GEB and other northern philanthropies between 1900 and 1930, see Eric Anderson and Alfred A. Moss Jr., *Dangerous Donations: Northern Philanthropy and Southern Black Education, 1902–1930* (Columbia: University of Missouri Press, 1999), 191–218.

57. "A Report of Conference on Child Welfare and Health Education Conducted by the School Health Coordinating Service in Cooperation with the North Carolina College for Negroes, June 7–July 17, 1940, by Walter J. Hughes, M.D.," General Education Board Records, Rockefeller Archive Center, North Tarrytown, New York, RG 1.3, ser. 950.4, box 542, folder 5815.

58. Paul B. Cornely to Walter Clarke, 22 April 1942, ASHA Papers, box 117, folder 6.

59. James H. Jones, *Bad Blood: The Tuskegee Syphilis Experiment—A Tragedy of Race and Medicine* (New York: Free Press, 1981).

60. Andrew J. Krog to Walter Clarke, 14 November 1944, ASHA Papers, box 118, folder 6.

61. Paul B. Cornely to Walter Clarke, 22 April 1942, Paul B. Cornely to Charles F. Marden, 7 September 1944, ASHA Papers, box 118, folder 7.

62. Esmond R. Long and Florence Seibert, "The Incidence of Tuberculosis Infection in American College Students," *Journal of the American Medical Association* 108 (1937): 1761–65; Esmond R. Long, "Tuberculosis in College Students, with Special Reference to Tuberculin Testing," *Journal-Lancet,* n.s. 55 (1937): 201–3; J. Arthur Meyers, "Types of Tuberculosis Lesions Found in the Chests of Students of Nursing and Medicine," *American Review of Tuberculosis* 28 (1933): 93–117.

63. For more on infection and mortality rates from tuberculosis during this period and the link between class and infection rates, see Barbara Bates, *Bargaining for Life: A Social History of Tuberculosis, 1876–1938* (Philadelphia: University of

Pennsylvania Press, 1992); Georgina D. Feldberg, *Disease and Class: Tuberculosis and the Shaping of North American Society* (New Brunswick, N.J.: Rutgers University Press, 1995); Barron H. Lerner, *Contagion and Confinement: Controlling Tuberculosis along the Skid Road* (Baltimore: Johns Hopkins University Press, 1998).

64. Martin S. Pernick, *The Black Stork: Eugenics and the Death of "Defective" Babies in American Medicine and Motion Pictures since 1915* (New York: Oxford University Press, 1996), 50–51 Barron H. Lerner, "Constructing Medical Indications: The Sterilization of Women with Heart Disease or Tuberculosis, 1905–1935," *Journal of the History of Medicine and Allied Sciences* 49, no. 3 (1994): 362–79.

65. Long, "Tuberculosis in College Students," 203.

66. Katherine Ott, *Fevered Lives: Tuberculosis in American Culture since 1870* (Cambridge: Harvard University Press, 1996), 148–49; Lerner, *Contagion and Confinement*, 31.

67. National Tuberculosis Association, *Tuberculosis and the 'Teen Age* (New York: National Tuberculosis Association, 1927).

68. Lee H. Ferguson, "Some Observations on Pulmonary Tuberculosis in Students," in *Proceedings of the American Student Health Association*, 1929, 48–49, American College Health Association Library, Linthicum, Maryland.

69. Edna Nicholson summarizes and criticizes these arguments about the causes of tuberculosis in women in *A Study of Tuberculosis Mortality among Young Women* (New York: National Tuberculosis Association, 1932), 8–9.

70. Glenadine Snow, "Health Problems of Women Students," in *Proceedings of the American Student Health Association*, 1925, 8–11, American College Health Association Library, Linthicum, Maryland; Ruby L. Cunningham, "Tuberculosis among University Women," *American Review of Tuberculosis* 31 (1935): 576–83.

71. Long and Seibert, "Incidence of Tuberculosis," 1765.

72. Long, "Tuberculosis in College Students," 201–4.

73. Long and Seibert, "Incidence of Tuberculosis," 1762–65.

74. National Tuberculosis Association, *Report of the Committee on Tuberculosis among Negroes* (New York: National Tuberculosis Association, 1937), 48–51.

75. Storey, *Status of Hygiene Programs*, 50, 114.

76. *Proceedings of the National Conference on College Hygiene* (New York: National Tuberculosis Association, 1931), 53–56.

77. Minutes of Executive Committee, American Student Health Association, 30 December 1931, ACHA Records, box 5, folder 10.

78. Lee H. Ferguson, "Pre-Symptom, Pre-Sign Tuberculosis in College Students," *Minutes and Proceedings of the Southern Student Health Association*, 4 June 1937, ACHA Records, box 4, folder 6.

79. Charles E. Shepard, "Campaign against Tuberculosis in College Students," *American Journal of Public Health* 25, no. 10 (1935): 1118.

80. Alfred Adler's work on the inferiority complex is best expressed in *The Neurotic Constitution: Outlines of a Comparative Individualistic Psychology and Psychotherapy*, trans. Bernard Glueck and John E. Lind (1926; Salem, N.H.: Ayer, 1983) and *The Practice and Theory of Individual Psychology*, trans. P. Radin (New York, Harcourt, Brace, 1932).

81. J. Arthur Meyers and L. M. Kernkamp, "Tuberculosis among Boys and

Girls in their Teens," *American Review of Tuberculosis* 21 (1930): 509–31; Stanley Gibson, "Athletic Activity at Puberty, with Special Reference to Cardiac and Tuberculosis Patients," *Journal of Pediatrics* 19 (1941): 382–86.

82. P. R. Hawley, "The Tuberculosis Problem of the Veterans' Administration," *American Review of Tuberculosis* 55 (1947): 1–7; Esmond R. Long, "The Tuberculosis Experience of the United States Army in World War II," *American Review of Tuberculosis* 55 (1947): 28–37.

83. Quoted in Jonathan Engel, *Doctors and Reformers: Discussion and Debate over Health Policy, 1925–1950* (Columbia: University of South Carolina Press, 2002), 230.

84. Harold S. Diehl and Charles E. Shepard, *The Health of College Students* (Washington, D.C.: American Council on Education, 1939), 44; Norman S. Moore and John Summerskill, *Health Services in American Colleges and Universities, 1953* (Ithaca: Cornell University Press, 1954).

85. President's Commission on Higher Education, *Higher Education for American Democracy*, vol. 1, *Establishing the Goals* (New York: Harper, 1948), 54.

86. Quoted in Dana L. Farnsworth, *College Health Services in the United States* (Student Personnel Series 4; Washington, D.C.: American College Personnel Association, 1965), 3.

87. Rickey Hendricks, *A Model for National Health Care: The History of Kaiser Permanente* (New Brunswick, N.J.: Rutgers University Press, 1993), 85–86.

88. Moore and Summerskill, *Health Services in American Colleges and Universities*, 23–25.

89. Ralph I. Canuteson, "College Self-Insurance Plans," in *Proceedings of the Thirty-first Annual Meeting of the American College Health Association*, 1953, 56–57.

90. Frank G. Dickinson and Everett L. Welker, *Second Survey of University and College Health Services: 1949–1950* (Chicago: American Medical Association, Bureau of Medical Economic Research, 1952), 4.

91. Quoted in Farnsworth, *College Health Services*, 4.

CHAPTER 6

1. Clifford Whittingham Beers, *A Mind That Found Itself: An Autobiography* (New York: Longmans, Green, 1908), 50–52; Norman Dain, *Clifford W. Beers: Advocate for the Insane* (Pittsburgh: University of Pittsburgh Press, 1980), 10–13.

2. Winifred Richmond, "Mental Hygiene in the Colleges," *Journal of the American Medical Association* 93 (1929): 1936.

3. A. M. Rossi, "Some Pre–World War II Antecedents of Community Mental Health Theory and Practice," *Mental Hygiene* 46 (1962): 78–98.

4. Jack Pressman, *Last Resort: Psychosurgery and the Limits of Medicine* (Cambridge: Cambridge University Press, 1998), 18–21.

5. Barbara Sicherman, *The Quest for Mental Health in America, 1880–1917* (New York: Arno, 1980), 421. See also Johannes Coenraad Pols, "Managing the Mind: The Culture of American Mental Hygiene, 1910–1950" (Ph.D. diss., University of Pennsylvania, 1997).

6. Arthur Hiler Ruggles, *Mental Health: Past, Present, and Future* (Providence, R.I.: Williams and Wilkins, 1934), 67–68.

7. Fred B. Rogers, "Stewart Paton (1865–1942): Mental Hygienist," *American Journal of Public Health* 55 (1965): 654–56.

8. Harry N. Kerns, "Cadet Problems," *Mental Hygiene* 7 (1923): 688–96.

9. Stewart Paton, *Education in War and Peace* (New York: Hoeber, 1920), vii, 71.

10. Lawrence J. Friedman, *Menninger: The Family and the Clinic* (Lawrence: University Press of Kansas, 1990), 33, 35; Karl A. Menninger, "Adaptation Difficulties in College Students," *Mental Hygiene* 11 (1927): 519.

11. Ernest Martin Hopkins to Stewart Paton, 14 April 1921, Arthur Hiler Ruggles to Ernest Martin Hopkins, 13 May 1913, President's Office Records, DP 11, box 36, folder 34, Rauner Special Collections Library, Dartmouth College, Hanover, New Hampshire.

12. A. F. Riggs and W. B. Terhune, "Mental Health of College Women," *Mental Hygiene* 12 (1928): 559–68. See also C. Mildred Thompson, "The Value of Mental Hygiene in the College," *Mental Hygiene* 11 (1927): 225–40.

13. Richmond, "Mental Hygiene in the Colleges," 1937; Florence Meredith, "The Administration of Mental Hygiene in Colleges," *Mental Hygiene* 11 (1927): 241–52.

14. M. C. Winternitz to Barry C. Smith, 15 January 1926, "Yale University—Department of Mental Hygiene," n.d., Commonwealth Fund Papers, RG 18.1, box 387, folder 3818, Rockefeller Archive Center, North Tarrytown, New York. For more on this subject, see J. W. Engel, "Early Psychiatry at Yale: Milton C. Winternitz and the Founding of the Department of Psychiatry and Mental Hygiene," *Yale Journal of Biology and Medicine* 67, nos. 1–2 (1994): 33–47.

15. Murray Levine and Julius Wishner, "The Case Records of the Psychological Clinic at the University of Pennsylvania," *Journal of the History of the Behavioral Sciences* 13, no. 1 (1977): 61.

16. Richmond, "Mental Hygiene in the Colleges," 1937; Sol Cohen, "The Mental Hygiene Movement and the Development of Personality: Changing Conceptions of the American College and University, 1920–1940," *History of Higher Education Annual* 2 (1982): 72.

17. Gerald Grob, *Mental Illness and American Society, 1875–1940* (Princeton: Princeton University Press, 1983); Elizabeth Lunbeck, *The Psychiatric Persuasion: Knowledge, Gender, and Power in Modern America* (Princeton: Princeton University Press, 1994).

18. Quoted in Sol Cohen, "Mental Hygiene Movement," 88.

19. Ernest Martin Hopkins to Mary Ross, 1 December 1924, President's Office Records, Dartmouth College, DP 11, folder 34, Mental Hygiene 1924–25.

20. Pernick, *Black Stork;* Digginbotham, *Keeping America Sane;* Zenderland, *Measuring Minds;* Kline, *Building a Better Race;* Stern, *Eugenic Nation.*

21. Nicolas Lemann, *The Big Test: The Secret History of American Meritocracy* (New York: Farrar, Straus, and Giroux, 1999).

22. Kathleen W. Jones, *Taming the Troublesome Child: American Families, Child Guidance, and the Limits of Psychiatric Authority* (Cambridge: Harvard University Press, 1999), 54.

23. Menninger, "Adaptation Difficulties," 519.

24. Marylynne Diggs, "Romantic Friends or a 'Different Race of Creatures'?

The Representation of Lesbian Pathology in Nineteenth Century America," *Feminist Studies* 21, no. 2 (1995): 317–40.

25. Quoted in Julia Grant, "A 'Real Boy' and Not a Sissy: Gender, Childhood, and Masculinity, 1890–1940," *Journal of Social History* 37, no. 4 (2004): 836. See also John C. Spurlock, "From Reassurance to Irrelevance: Adolescent Psychology and Homosexuality in America," *History of Psychology* 5, no. 1 (2002): 38–51.

26. Kerns, "Cadet Problems," 690, 693–94. See also Harry N. Kerns, "Management of Acute Mental-Hygiene Problems," *Mental Hygiene* 9 (1925): 273–81.

27. Kathleen W. Jones, "Suicide, 'Faggoty Parties,' and Harvard's Secret Disciplinary Court: Homosexual Panic in 1920," paper presented at the annual meeting of the Society for History of Childhood and Youth, Milwaukee, Wisconsin, August 2005.

28. Jerome Karabel, *The Chosen: The Hidden History of Admission and Exclusion at Harvard, Yale, and Princeton* (New York: Houghton Mifflin, 2005), 83, 106–8, 119.

29. Charles W. Burr, "Broken Minds of Youth," *Hygeia* 6 (1928): 547–48.

30. Quoted in Kathleen W. Jones, *Taming the Troublesome Child*, 112. For a fuller discussion of anti-Semitism and homophobia in the trial, see Paul B. Franklin, "Jew Boys, Queer Boys: Rhetorics of Antisemitism and Homophobia in the Trial of Nathan 'Babe' Leopold, Jr. and Richard 'Dickie' Loeb," in *Queer Theory and the Jewish Question*, ed. Daniel Boyarin, Daniel Itzkovitz, and Ann Pellegrini (New York: Columbia University Press, 2003), 121–48. See also Paula S. Fass, "Making and Remaking an Event: The Leopold and Loeb Case in American Culture," *Journal of American History* 80, no. 3 (1993): 919–51.

31. Thompson, "Value of Mental Hygiene," 236–37.

32. Meredith, "Administration of Mental Hygiene," 251.

33. Quoted in Crista Jean Deluzio, "'New Girls for Old': Female Adolescence in American Scientific Thought, 1870–1930" (Ph.D. diss., Brown University, 1999), 294–96.

34. Milton Wittler to Mary Ware Dennett, 13 December 1933, Annie R. Dyer to Mary Ware Dennett, n.d., Eric Thomson to Mary Ware Dennett, 30 May 1928, Mary Ware Dennett Papers, MC 392/M-138, reel 25, Schlesinger Library, Radcliffe Institute for Advanced Study, Cambridge, Massachusetts. There collection contains numerous other faculty requests for copies of the pamphlet.

35. Fass, *Damned and the Beautiful;* Bailey, *From Front Porch to Back Seat;* Horowitz, *Campus Life.*

36. Exner, "College and Social Hygiene Education," 30.

37. Clement Fry and Edna G. Rostow, *Mental Health in College* (New York: Commonwealth Fund, 1942), 4–5, 18, 8–9.

38. "Retrospect and Prospect: A Special Report on the Twenty-fifth Anniversary of the Student Mental Hygiene Service at Yale, June 1951," Clement Fry Papers, box 3, Manuscripts and Archives Division, Sterling Library, Yale University, New Haven, Connecticut.

39. "Prospectus for a Program of Studies in the Emotional and Social Problems of Youth, 1945," Records of the Department of University Health, Division of Student Mental Hygiene, box 10, folder 39, Manuscripts and Archives Division, Sterling Library, Yale University, New Haven, Connecticut.

40. William C. Menninger, introduction to *The Story of GAP*, by Albert Deutsch (New York: Group for the Advancement of Psychiatry, 1959), 3–4.

41. Deutsch, *The Story of GAP*, 7–8.

42. President's Commission on Higher Education, *Higher Education for American Democracy*, 53–54.

43. Dana Farnsworth and Augustus Thorndike, "Medical Progress: Health in Colleges and Universities," *New England Journal of Medicine* 255, no. 20 (1956): 950; Dana Farnsworth and Augustus Thorndike, "Medical Progress: Health in Colleges and Universities (Concluded)," *New England Journal of Medicine* 255, no. 21 (1956): 993.

44. Clement Fry to Dana Farnsworth, 9 March 1945, Dana Farnsworth to Clement Fry, 27 March 1945, Records of the Department of University Health, Division of Student Mental Hygiene, Yale University, box 21, folder 62.

45. William C. Menninger to Clement Fry, 23 March 1948, Records of the Department of University Health, Division of Student Mental Hygiene, Yale University, box 13, folder 84.

46. Group for the Advancement of Psychiatry, Committee on Academic Education, *The Role of Psychiatrists in Colleges and Universities* (New York: Group for the Advancement of Psychiatry, 1951), 1, 5.

47. Group for the Advancement of Psychiatry, Committee on the College Student, *Considerations on Personality Development in College Students* (Topeka, Kans.: Group for the Advancement of Psychiatry, 1955), 1–2.

48. Beth Bailey, *Sex in the Heartland* (Cambridge: Harvard University Press, 1999), 84–85.

49. Jonathan Zimmerman, "'One's Total World View Comes into Play': America's Culture War over Alcohol Education, 1945–1964," *History of Education Quarterly* 42, no. 4 (2002): 471–92.

50. Ernest Martin Hopkins to Doctor Baketel, 2 January 1918, President's Office Records, Dartmouth College, DP 11, box 15, FF 105.

51. Zimmerman, "'One's Total World View."

52. Sarah W. Tracy, *Alcoholism in America: From Reconstruction to Prohibition* (Baltimore: Johns Hopkins University Press, 2004), 281–82.

53. Clement Fry, "Drinking in College," *Hygeia* 26 (1948): 710–11.

54. "Seminar, Problems of Yale Student Drinking," 17 April 1951, Records of the Department of University Health, Division of Student Mental Hygiene, Yale University, box 1, folder 3.

55. Robert Straus and Selden Bacon, *Drinking in College* (New Haven: Yale University Press, 1953), 37, 41, 44.

56. Ibid., 211–12.

57. Alfred C. Kinsey, *Sexual Behavior in the Human Male* (Philadelphia: Saunders, 1948); Alfred C. Kinsey, *Sexual Behavior in the Human Female* (Philadelphia: Saunders, 1953).

58. Straus and Bacon, *Drinking in College*, 187–88.

59. Fry and Rostow, *Mental Health in College*, 8–9.

60. "Notes on Seminar: Problems of the Yale Student—Drinking," 20 March 1951, Records of the Department of University Health, Division of Student Mental Hygiene, Yale University, box 1, folder 3.

61. Henry Harper Hart, "Fear of Homosexuality in College Students," in *Psychosocial Problems of College Men*, ed. Bryan M. Wedge (New Haven: Yale University Press, 1958), 200, 213.

62. Everett Hunt, "The Dean and the Psychiatrist," *Mental Hygiene* 37 (1953), 187–88.

63. Bailey, *Sex in the Heartland*, 86–90.

64. Dana L. Farnsworth, "College Health Comes of Age," *Journal-Lancet* 74, no. 10 (1954): 397–401.

65. Ethel L. Ginsburg, *The College and Student Health* (New York: National Tuberculosis Association, 1955), 46–48.

CHAPTER 7

1. Marvin Harris, "Big Bust on Morningside Heights," *Nation*, 10 June 1968, 757.

2. "Couch on Campus: Psychiatric Experts Find Danger in Bright, Immature Students," *New York Times*, 26 April 1964, E9.

3. "Students Comment," *Vassar Miscellany News*, 11 April 1962, 2.

4. Dana L. Farnsworth, "College Mental Health and Social Change," *Annals of Internal Medicine* 73, no. 3 (1970): 470.

5. "Couch on Campus."

6. Robert Coles and Joseph Brenner, "American Youth in a Social Struggle: The Mississippi Summer Project," *American Journal of Orthopsychiatry* 35, no. 5 (1965): 909–26.

7. Quoted in W. J. Rorabaugh, *Berkeley at War: The 1960s* (New York: Oxford University Press, 1989), 22.

8. "Twenty at Yale Fined in Morals Case; 8 Still in School to Be Expelled," *New York Times*, 28 January 1960, 22.

9. Robert L. Arnstein, "Sex and Anxiety on the Campus: Thirty-five Years Thereof," *Journal of American College Health* 37, no. 6 (1989): 248–49.

10. "Seminar—Problems of the Yale Student—The Homosexual within the Community," 12 February 1952, Records of the Department of University Health, Division of Student Mental Hygiene, Yale University, box 1, folder 3.

11. Arnstein, "Sex and Anxiety on the Campus," 247.

12. Group for the Advancement of Psychiatry, Committee on the College Student, *Sex and the College Student* (New York: Group for the Advancement of Psychiatry, 1965), 10, 44, 98–99.

13. *Griswold v. Connecticut*, 381 U.S. 479 (1965). For more on the evolution of the concept of the right to privacy in American jurisprudence, see David J. Garrow, *Liberty and Sexuality: The Right to Privacy and the Making of* Roe v. Wade (Berkeley: University of California Press, 1998); John W. Johnson, Griswold v. Connecticut: *Birth Control and the Constitutional Right of Privacy* (Lawrence: University Press of Kansas, 2005).

14. *Eisenstadt v. Baird*, 405 U.S. 438 (1972).

15. Harriet F. Pilpel and Nancy F. Wechsler, "Birth Control, Teenagers, and the Law," *Family Planning Perspectives* 1, no. 1 (1969): 29–35.

16. Group for the Advancement of Psychiatry, Committee on the College Student, *Sex and the College Student*, 105.

17. "The Pill on Campus," *Newsweek*, 11 October 1965, 92–93.

18. "Brown Backs Doctor on Birth Control Pills," *Providence (Rhode Island) Journal*, 29 September 1965. Clipping from Brown University Archives.

19. "Pill on Campus," 93.

20. Philip M. Sarrel and Lorna J. Sarrel, "Birth Control Services and Sex Counseling at Yale," *Family Planning Perspectives* 3, no. 3 (1971): 33.

21. "Brown's Birth Pill Incident under Fire," *Boston Globe*, 29 September 1965. Clipping from Brown University Archives.

22. Robert Gage, interview, in David Cline, *Creating Choice: A Community Responds to the Need for Abortion and Birth Control, 1961–1973* (New York: Palgrave, 2006), 87.

23. "L.I. Man Arrested while Distributing Birth-Control Data," *New York Times*, 14 May 1965, 22.

24. A. Goldberg, "The Perils of the Pill," *Ramparts*, May 1969, 45–48.

25. Natalie Jaffe, "Campus on L.I. Gets Birth-Curb Group," *New York Times*, 27 March 1966, 66.

26. Goldberg, "The Perils of the Pill," 45–46.

27. Beverly Eschenburg, "Bill Baird: Betrayed?" *Kaleidoscope*, June 1970, 11.

28. "Birth-Control Ban Protested by Pickets at St. Patrick's," *New York Times*, 13 August 1966, 12.

29. Linda Thurston, *Birth Control, Abortion, and Venereal Disease* (Cambridge, Mass.: Resist, 1970).

30. Pamela Swift, "Student Sex Clinics," *Philadelphia Sunday Bulletin*, 29 August 1971, clipping from Radcliffe Archives News Office, RG X, ser. 7, box 27, folder 406, Schlesinger Library, Radcliffe Institute for Advanced Study, Cambridge, Massachusetts.

31. Larry Berger, "Student Guide for Birth Control, Abortion, VD, and Drugs: Resources in the Boston Area," 1970, Boston Women's Health Book Collective Papers, ser. II, box 1, folders 1.13–1.14, Schlesinger Library, Radcliffe Institute for Advanced Study, Cambridge, Massachusetts.

32. Copies of these and other manuals are contained in the Takey Crist Papers, box 27, Special Collections, Sallie Bingham Center for Women's History and Culture, Duke University. For a review of these books, see Takey Crist and Lana Starnes, "Review: Student Printing Presses Bring Birth Control Story to Colleges," *Family Planning Perspectives* 4, no. 1 (1972): 60–61.

33. Henry Woodhead, "At 20, He Teaches 'That Course,'" *Daily Tar Heel*, ca. 1970, Crist Papers, box 21.

34. James Trussell and Steve Chandler, *The Loving Book* (Charlotte, N.C.: Red Clay, 1971). For more on the Institute for the Study of Health and Society, see Naomi Rogers, "'Caution: The AMA May Be Dangerous to Your Health': The Student Health Organizations (SHO) and American Medicine, 1965–1970," *Radical History Review* 80 (2001) 5–34.

35. Swift, "Student Sex Clinics."

36. "Contraceptive Counseling, Classes on Sex Seen Needed on Campus," *Ob. Gyn. News*, 1 May 1970, 6.

37. Walker Lundy, "Never Have So Many Been So Unabashed: U-M Meets Sex Problem Head On," *Detroit Free Press*, 8 April 1969; Linda Quinet, "Marguerite Shearer," n.d., University Health Service Records, University of Michigan, box 4, scrapbook.

38. Swift, "Student Sex Clinics."

39. Martin Gansberg, "150 Fordham Women Petition for a Class on Birth Control," *New York Times*, 7 May 1967, 41.

40. Sarrel and Sarrel, "Birth Control Services and Sex Counseling," 33.

41. "Should Colleges Set Up Campus Birth-Control Clinics?" *Glamour*, February 1970, 206.

42. Takey Crist, telephone interview by author, 21 October 2006.

43. Andrew Malcolm, "What They Don't Know about Sex," *New York Times*, 15 August 1971, clipping, Crist Papers, box 5.

44. "The Pill at Stanford," *Time*, 28 November 1969, accessed online 9 April 2007.

45. Eugene Schoenfeld, *Doctor Hip Pocrates: Advice Your Family Doctor Never Gave You* (New York: Grove, 1969).

46. "Birth Control Info at Cowell," *Daily Californian*, 30 September 1965, 2.

47. "Should Colleges Set Up Campus Birth-Control Clinics?"

48. "No Birth Control," *Daily Californian*, 3 February 1967, 3.

49. Program Description, Planned Parenthood–World Population College Programs, Sophia Smith Collection, Smith College, Northampton, Massachusetts, (hereafter cited as PPFA II Papers), box 56, folder 11.

50. Dan Pellegrom to Douglas Stewart, 30 September 1969, PPFA II Papers, box 56, folder 1.

51. Samuel Taylor to Douglas Stewart, 27 March 1969, PPFA II Papers, box 56, folder 1.

52. "A Program of Student Community Action (A Working Document) for Planned Parenthood—World Population," June 1969, PPFA II Papers, box 56, folder 1.

53. Dan Pellegrom to Doug Stewart, 30 September 1969, PPFA II Papers, box 56, folder 1.

54. Roy Beck and Leon Kolankiewicz, "The Environmental Movement's Retreat from Advocating U.S. Population Stabilization (1970–1998): A First Draft of History," *Journal of Policy History* 12, no. 1 (2000): 123–56.

55. Takey Crist and Lana Starnes, "Sex Books on the Campus—A New Plea for Old Information. Points to Ponder," typescript, n.d., Crist Papers, box 5.

56. Dan Pellegrom to Nancy Clark, 6 January 1969, 28 January 1970, PPFA II Papers, box 55, folder 87.

57. Dan Pellegrom to Michael Metcalf, 23 January 1970, PPFA II Papers, box 55, folder 87.

58. Naomi Gray to Douglas Stewart, 30 September 1969, PPFA II Papers, box 56, folder 1.

59. Ethel M. Nash, "The College Physician's Role in Sex Education," *Journal of the American College Health Association* 15, supplement (1967): 69.

60. Mary Smith, "Birth Control Pills and the Negro Woman," *Ebony*, 23 March 1968, 34. For more on the issue of birth control and black allegations of

genocide, see Simone M. Caron, "Birth Control and the Black Community in the 1960s: Genocide or Power Politics?" *Journal of Social History* 31, no. 3 (1998): 545–59.

61. Woodhead, "At 20, He Teaches 'That Course.'"

62. Donna Cherniak and Allan Feingold, *The Birth Control Handbook*, 4th ed., rev. (Montreal: Journal Offset, 1970). For more on the birth control movement at Canadian colleges and universities, see Christabelle Sethna, "The University of Toronto Health Service, Oral Contraception, and Student Demand for Birth Control, 1960–1970," *Historical Studies in Education* 17, no. 2 (2005): 265–92; Christabelle Sethna, "The Evolution of the *Birth Control Handbook:* From Student Peer Education Manual to Feminist Self-Help Text, 1968–1975," *Canadian Bulletin of Medical History* 23, no. 1 (2006): 89–117.

63. Alan F. Guttmacher and Gene Vadies, "Sex on the Campus and the College Health Service," paper presented at the annual meeting of the American College Health Association, Atlanta, 6 April 1972, PPFA II Papers, box 56, folder 15.

64. "Should Colleges Set Up Campus Birth-Control Clinics?"

65. Guttmacher and Vadies, "Sex on the Campus."

66. *Eisenstadt v. Baird*, 405 U.S. 438 (1972).

67. Thomas S. Szasz, "The Psychiatrist as Double Agent," *Trans-Action* 15, no. 1 (1967): 18–24; Thomas S. Szasz, "College Psychiatry: A Critique," *Comprehensive Psychiatry* 9, no. 1 (1968): 81–85.

68. Dana L. Farnsworth, "Student Unrest and the College Health Service," *Journal of the American College Health Association* 18, no. 2 (1969): 125–26.

69. Robert L. Arnstein, "The College Mental Health Practitioner as Change Agent," *Journal of the American College Health Association* 25, no. 3 (1977): 198–99.

70. Robert L. Arnstein, "Patient Rights: The Yale Experience," *Journal of the American College Health Association* 27, no. 3 (1978): 132–33.

71. Ibid., 133, 169.

72. Dana L. Farnsworth, "College Dropouts," *Rhode Island Medical Journal* 52, no. 1 (1969): 210.

73. David E. Smith, "Runaways and Their Health Problems in Haight-Ashbury during the Summer of 1967," *American Journal of Public Health* 59, no. 11 (1969): 2046–47. See also David E. Smith, *Love Needs Care: A History of San Francisco's Haight-Ashbury Free Medical Clinic* (Boston: Little, Brown, 1971); Richard B. Seymour and David E. Smith, *The Haight-Ashbury Free Medical Clinics: Still Free after All These Years, 1967–1987* (San Francisco: Partisan, 1986).

74. Joseph Brenner, "A Free Clinic for Medical Care," *New York Times Magazine*, 11 October 1970, 30–31, 107–17; Joseph Brenner, interview by author, 19 February 1991; Parker Donham, "Doctors to Establish Free Clinic," *Harvard Crimson*, 29 November 1967, accessed online 9 April 2007.

75. Herbert J. Freudenberger and Arlene P. Freudenberger, *1973—The Free Clinic Picture Today—A Survey* (New York: American Psychological Association, 1974). For more on the free clinic movement in Canada, see Carrie Dickenson, "No Place Like Home: Canada and the Response to the Transient Youth Phenomenon, 1960–1980," Ph.D. diss., McMaster University, forthcoming.

76. "Student Health Service Committee," *Daily Californian*, 6 April 1965, 6; "Cowell Psyc Center Rapped," *Daily Californian*, 15 April 1971, 8.

77. Henry Bruyn, Edna Brean, Lucile Withington, Karen Topp Goodwyn, Gerald Belchick, and John Velton. interviews conducted as part of Disability Rights and Independent Living Movement Oral History Series, 1994–98, available online at http://ark.cdlib.org/ark:/13030/kt5z09n82q, accessed 7 March 2007; Larry A. Biscamp to Rod Carter, 18 September 1969, Disabled Students Program, CU 479, carton 1, folder 11, Bancroft Library, University of California, Berkeley; Toni Martin, "Students Denounce Cowell," *Daily Californian*, 23 April 1971, 1.

78. "Coalition Handbook," *Daily Tar Heel*, 8 April 1975.

79. Robert W. Gage, "The President's Message," *American College Health Association Newsletter* 12, no. 3 (1970): 1–2.

80. Kent E. Robinson, "The Attack on Student Services," *New Directions for Higher Education* 1, no. 3 (1973): 1–4. For more on Bruyn's resignation from Berkeley, see Bruyn, interview, Disability Rights and Independent Living Movement Oral History.

81. Lisa Culberson and Beth Rosenberg, "Students Complain Health Service Slow," *Michigan Daily*, 4 February 1978, University Health Service Records, University of Michigan, box 4.

82. "Former Student to Head Cowell," *Daily Californian*, 16 April 1973, 7; "Little Known Service: Free Abortions Given at Cowell," *Daily Californian*, 5 February 1974, 1; Andrew E. Wade, "Student Consumer Rights," *Daily Californian*, 14 October 1974, 5.

83. J. B. Kelly to trustees, 22 August 1979, Kathleen Pointer to trustees, 22 August 1979, Student Health Service Records, box 1, University Archives, Wilson Library, University of North Carolina at Chapel Hill.

84. Memo re: ACHA, 26 February 1974, "Discussion with Dr. Samuel I. Fuenning, Director and Professor, Nebraska Center for Health Education, University of Nebraska, and Dr. J. Lawrence Manuell, Director, University Health Service, New York University, concerning the ACHA. Present Dr. Fitz and Mr. Donway," 17 February 1976, Commonwealth Fund Papers.

85. Quoted in H. Spencer Turner and Janet L. Hurley, *The History and Practice of College Health* (Lexington: University Press of Kentucky, 2002), 14.

86. Theodore R. Marmor, "The Politics of Universal Health Insurance: Lessons from the Past?" *Journal of Interdisciplinary History* 26, no. 4 (1996): 671–79.

87. H. Spencer Turner, "New Realities: The Challenge to Change," *Journal of the American College Health Association* 30, no. 1 (1981): 7–9.

CHAPTER 8

1. Richard P. Keeling, "College Health Responds to HIV: Hard Lessons and a Rich Heritage," *Journal of American College Health* 43, no. 6 (1995): 271.

2. Richard P. Keeling, "AIDS on the College Campus: Introduction," *Journal of American College Health* 35, no. 3 (1986): 123–26.

3. "Editorial: AIDS and the College Health Service," *Journal of American College Health* 35, no. 3 (1986): 122.

4. National Student Association, *Gays on Campus* (Washington, D.C.: National Student Association, 1975), 7.

5. Patrick Dilley, *Gay Man on Campus: A History of Non-Heterosexual College Men, 1945–2000* (New York: Routledge Falmer, 2002), 173–75.

6. "Students Run Stanford AIDS Education Project," *Advocate*, 16 September 1986, 17.

7. Cathy Kodama and Mary O'Donnell, *AIDS Education on the College Campus: A Practical Guide* (Berkeley: Health Promotion Office, University of California, 1987), 3–7.

8. Toby Simon, "Sexuality on Campus—'90s Style," *Change* 25 (1993): 50.

9. Richard P. Keeling, "HIV/AIDS: The Once and Future Epidemic," 2003, available online at www.keelingassociates.com, accessed 13 July 2006.

10. Simon, "Sexuality on Campus"; Alex P. Kellogg, "'Safe Sex Fatigue' Grows among Gay Students," *Chronicle of Higher Education*, 18 January 2002, A37; Leo Reisberg, "Colleges Start Clinics for Doctor-Averse Men," *Chronicle of Higher Education*, 7 July 2000, A7.

11. Jeffrey Young, "Prozac Campus: More Students Seek Counseling and Take Psychiatric Medication," *Chronicle of Higher Education*, 13 February 2003, A37–38.

12. Richard Kadison and Theresa Foy Digeronimo, *College of the Overwhelmed: The Campus Mental Health Crisis and What to Do about It* (San Francisco: Jossey-Bass, 2004), 153.

13. American College Health Association, "American College Health Association National College Health Assessment Spring 2006 Reference Group Data Report (Abridged)," *Journal of American College Health* 55, no. 4 (January–February 2007): 204–5.

14. Robert B. Smith and Dana L. Fleming, "Student Suicide and Colleges' Liability," *Chronicle of Higher Education*, 20 April 2007, B24; Tamar Lewin, "Laws Limit Options when a Student Is Mentally Ill," *New York Times*, 19 April 2007, 1.

15. Kevin Patrick, "The History and Current Status of College Health," in *Principles and Practice of Student Health*, vol. 3, *College Health*, ed. Helen M. Wallace et al. (Oakland, Calif.: Third Party, 1992), 508–9.

16. Lynn Love, "Just What the Doctor Ordered," *University Business* 2, no. 4 (1999): 25–29.

17. Eric Wills, "Parent Trap," *Chronicle of Higher Education*, 22 July 2005, A4; Helen E. Johnson, "Educating Parents about College Life," *Chronicle of Higher Education*, 9 January 2004, B11; Wendy White, "Students, Parents, Colleges: Drawing the Lines," *Chronicle of Higher Education*, 16 December 2005, B16.

18. Paula S. Fass, *Outside In: Minorities and the Transformation of American Education* (New York: Oxford University Press, 1989), 3–4.

19. Timothy M. Osberg, "A Business Case for Increasing College Mental Health Services," *Behavioral Health Management*, September–October 2004, 33–36.

20. Richard P. Keeling, "Drinking in College: The Politics of Research and Prevention," *Journal of American College Health* 47, no. 2 (1998): 51–55.

21. Lawrence Neinstein, *The Healthy Student: A Parent's Guide to Preparing Teens for the College Years* (Blue Hills, Mo.: Society for Adolescent Medicine, 2003), available online at http://www.adolescenthealth.org/The_Healthy_Student.pdf, accessed 13 July 2006.

22. *Student Health Spectrum*, June 2004, available online at http://www.chickering.com/spectrum/archives.aspx, accessed 19 July 2006.

23. Association of American Colleges and Universities, Program for Health and Higher Education, available online at http://www.aacu-edu.org/phhe/overview/index.cfm, accessed 13 July 2006.

Selected Bibliography

MANUSCRIPT COLLECTIONS

American College Health Association Library, Linthicum, Maryland

ACHA Executive Committee Meetings Record Books
ACHA *Transactions*
Proceedings of the American Student Health Association

Amherst College Archives and Special Collections, Amherst, Massachusetts

Edward (AC 1849) and Mary Judson Hitchcock Papers
Papers Connected with the Department of Physical Education

College of Physicians of Philadelphia Historical Library, Philadelphia

S. Weir Mitchell Papers

Cornell University, Division of Rare Books and Manuscripts, Ithaca, New York

Andrew Dickson White Papers
Typhoid Fever Epidemic (Ithaca, NY) Records, 1901–1906

Dartmouth College, Rauner Special Collections Library, Hanover, New Hampshire

Isolation Hospital Log Books
President's Office Records

Duke University, Special Collections, Sallie Bingham Center for Women's History and Culture, Durham, North Carolina

Takey Crist Papers

Harvard University Archives, Cambridge, Massachusetts

President's Annual Reports
Dudley Allen Sargent Papers

Howard University Archives, Washington, D.C.

Dorothy Boulding Ferebee Papers

Ithaca City Hall, Ithaca, New York

Minutes of the Board of Health

National Library of Medicine, Bethesda, Maryland

Paul Bertau Cornely Papers
Louis I. Dublin Papers

Rockefeller Archive Center, North Tarrytown, New York

Bureau of Social Hygiene
Commonwealth Fund Papers
General Education Board, New Southern Program
Office of Mssrs. Rockefeller

Schlesinger Library, Radcliffe Institute for Advanced Study, Cambridge, Massachusetts

Boston Women's Health Book Collective Papers
Class of 1899 Collections
Mary Ware Dennett Papers
Radcliffe College Annual Reports

Smith College, Sophia Smith Collection, Northampton, Massachusetts

Planned Parenthood Federation of America Records

Stanford University Special Collections, Stanford, California

American Student Health Association Papers
Clelia Duel Mosher Papers
Thomas A. Storey Papers
Student Guild Records

University of California, Berkeley, Bancroft Library

Board of Regents Records
Disabled Students Program
Office of the President, University Board of Health Records

University of Michigan, Bentley Historical Library, Ann Arbor

Eliza Mosher Papers
John Sundwall Papers
University Health Service Records

University of Minnesota, Andersen Library, Minneapolis

University Archives
Board of Regents Minutes
Ruth Evelyn Boynton Papers
University Health Service Records

Social Welfare History Archives
American Social Hygiene Association Papers

University of North Carolina, Chapel Hill, University Archives, Wilson Library
Student Health Service Records

University of Pennsylvania Archives, Philadelphia
R. Tait McKenzie Papers

Yale University, Manuscripts and Archives Division, Sterling Library, New Haven, Connecticut
Isidore S. Falk Papers
Clement Fry Papers
Records of the Department of University Health, Division of Student Mental Hygiene

PUBLISHED PRIMARY SOURCES

Adams, Samuel Hopkins. "Typhoid: An Unnecessary Evil." *McClure's*, June 1905, 145, 150–52.

Adler, Alfred. *The Neurotic Constitution: Outlines of a Comparative Individualistic Psychology and Psychotherapy*. Trans. Bernard Glueck and John E. Lind. 1926. Salem, N.H.: Ayer, 1983.

Adler, Alfred. *The Practice and Theory of Individual Psychology*. Trans. P. Radin. New York: Harcourt, Brace, 1932.

Allen, Nathan. *Changes in New England Population*. Lowell, Mass.: Stone, Huse, 1877.

Allen, Nathan. *The Education of Girls, as Connected with Their Growth and Development*. Boston: Bicknell, 1879.

Allen, Nathan. *Physical Culture in Amherst College*. Lowell, Mass.: Stone and Huse, 1869.

American Medical Association, Bureau of Medical Economics. *University and College Health Centers*. Chicago: American Medical Association, 1936.

Arnstein, Robert L. "The College Mental Health Practitioner as Change Agent?" *Journal of the American College Health Association* 25, no. 3 (1977): 198–200.

Arnstein, Robert L. "Patient Rights: The Yale Experience." *Journal of the American College Health Association* 27, no. 3 (1978): 132–33, 169.

Arnstein, Robert L. "Sex and Anxiety on the Campus: Thirty-five Years Thereof." *Journal of American College Health* 37, no. 6 (1989): 247–53.

Baer, Clara Gregory. "Health of College Women." In *Proceedings of the National Education Association of the United States*, 1916, 690–93.

Beers, Clifford Whittingham. *A Mind That Found Itself: An Autobiography*. New York: Longmans, Green, 1908.

Bowles, Gordon T. *New Types of Old Americans at Harvard and at Eastern Women's Colleges*. Cambridge: Harvard University Press, 1932.

Brackett, Anna C., ed. *Education of American Girls, Considered in a Series of Essays*. New York: Putnam, 1874.

Canuteson, Ralph I. "College Self-Insurance Plans." *Proceedings of the Thirty-first Annual Meeting of the American College Health Association*, 1953, 56–57.

Clarke, Edward H. *Sex in Education; or, A Fair Chance for the Girls*. Boston: Osgood, 1873.

Coles, Robert, and Joseph Brenner. "American Youth in a Social Struggle: The Mississippi Summer Project." *American Journal of Orthopsychiatry* 35, no. 5 (1965): 909–27.

Cook, C. H. "The Effect of College Life at Wellesley." *Medical Communications of the Massachusetts Medical Society* 16 (1893): 191–95.

Cornely, Paul B. "Health Education—An Urgent Need in Negro Colleges." *National Negro Health Newsletter* 8, no. 2 (1940): 11–14.

Cornely, Paul B. "Health Education Programs in Negro Colleges." *Journal of Negro Education* 6, no. 3 (1937): 531–37.

Cornely, Paul B. "The Status of Student Health Programs in Negro Colleges in 1938–39." *Journal of Negro Education* 10, no. 2 (1941): 151–67.

Crist, Takey, and Lana Starnes. "Review: Student Printing Presses Bring Birth Control Story to Colleges." *Family Planning Perspectives* 4, no. 1 (1972): 60–61.

Cunningham, Ruby L. "Tuberculosis among University Women." *American Review of Tuberculosis* 31 (1935): 576–83.

Davis, Katherine Bement. *Factors in the Sex Life of Twenty-two Hundred Women.* New York: Harper, 1929.

Dickinson, Frank G., and Everett L. Welker. *Second Survey of University and College Health Services: 1949–1950.* Chicago: American Medical Association, Bureau of Medical Economic Research, 1952.

Diehl, Harold S. "Health Exams for College Students." *Hygeia* 8 (1930): 51–54.

Diehl, Harold S., and Charles E. Shepard. *The Health of College Students.* Washington, D.C.: American Council on Education, 1939.

Dublin, Louis I. "The Significance of the Declining Birth Rate." *Science,* 1 March 1918, 201–10.

Earp, J. Rosslyn. "Hygiene in an American College." *Hygeia* 2 (1924): 613–14.

Eliot, Charles W. "The American Social Hygiene Association." *Journal of Social Hygiene* 1, no. 1 (1914): 1–5.

Exner, Max J. "The College and Social Hygiene Education." *Proceedings of the Sixth Annual Meeting of the American Student Health Association,* 1925, 23–30.

Exner, Max J. "Sex Education by the Young Men's Christian Association in Universities and Colleges." *Journal of Social Hygiene* 1, no. 4 (1915): 570–80.

Farnsworth, Dana L. "College Health Comes of Age." *Journal-Lancet* 74, no. 10 (1954): 397–401.

Farnsworth, Dana L. *College Health Services in the United States.* Student Personnel Series 4. Washington, D.C.: American College Personnel Association, 1965.

Farnsworth, Dana L. *Mental Health in College and University.* Cambridge: Harvard University Press, 1957.

Farnsworth, Dana L. "Student Unrest and the College Health Service." *Journal of the American College Health Association* 18, no. 2 (1969): 125–30.

Ferguson, Lee H. "Some Observations on Pulmonary Tuberculosis in Students." *Proceedings of the American Student Health Association,* 1929, 48–49.

Forsythe, Warren E. "Health Service in American Colleges and Universities." *Journal of the American Medical Association* 63, no. 22 (1914): 1926–30.

Forsythe, Warren E. *Health Service in American Colleges and Universities.* Ann Arbor: University of Michigan, 1926.

Forsythe, Warren E. "Student Health Work." *School and Society* 4 (1916): 439–44.

Freudenberger, Herbert J., and Arlene P. Freudenberger. *1973—The Free Clinic Picture Today—A Survey.* New York: American Psychological Association, 1974.

Fry, Clement, and Edna G. Rostow. *Mental Health in College.* New York: Commonwealth Fund, 1942.

Gibson, Stanley "Athletic Activity at Puberty, with Special Reference to Cardiac and Tuberculosis Patients." *Journal of Pediatrics* 19 (1941): 382–86.

Ginsburg, Ethel L. *The College and Student Health.* New York: National Tuberculosis Association, 1955.

Gordon, Faith Fairfield. "Physical Measurements of One Thousand Smith College Students." *American Journal of Public Health* 20, no. 9 (1930): 963–68.

Griswold Don M., and Hazel I. Spicer. *University Student Health Services.* Publications of the Committee on the Costs of Medical Care 19. Chicago: University of Chicago Press, 1932.

Group for the Advancement of Psychiatry, Committee on Academic Education. *The Role of Psychiatrists in Colleges and Universities.* New York: Group for the Advancement of Psychiatry, 1951.

Group for the Advancement of Psychiatry, Committee on the College Student. *Considerations on Personality Development in College Students.* Topeka, Kans.: Group for the Advancement of Psychiatry, 1955.

Group for the Advancement of Psychiatry, Committee on the College Student. *Sex and the College Student.* New York: Group for the Advancement of Psychiatry, 1965.

Hall, G. Stanley. *Adolescence: Its Psychology and Its Relation to Physiology, Anthropology, Sociology, Sex, Crime, Religion, and Education.* New York: Appleton, 1904.

Hall, G. Stanley. "Student Customs." *Proceedings of the American Antiquarian Society,* n.s. 14 (1900): 83–124.

Hall, G. Stanley. "The Teaching of Sex in Schools and Colleges." *Social Diseases* 2, no. 4 (1911): 1–19.

Hartley, Sophie M. "The Influence of Higher Education upon Women with Reference to Their Ability to Propagate Healthy Species." *Woman's Medical Journal* 4 (1895): 319–21.

Hartwell, Edward M. *Physical Training in American Colleges and Universities.* Washington, D.C.: U.S. Government Printing Office, 1885.

Hawley, P. R. "The Tuberculosis Problem of the Veterans' Administration." *American Review of Tuberculosis* 55 (1947): 1–7.

Henderson, Rose. "Colleges and Health." *Hygeia* 11 (1933): 777–79.

Hitchcock, Edward, Jr. "The Department of Physical Education and Hygiene in Amherst College." *Massachusetts State Board of Health Reports* 10 (1879): 63–72.

Hitchcock, Edward, Jr. "Hygiene at Amherst College." *American Public Health Association Papers and Reports* 4 (1877–78): 46–56.

Hitchcock, Edward, Jr. *A Report of Twenty Years Experience in the Department of Physical Education at Amherst College.* Amherst, Mass.: Bangs, 1881.

Howe, Julia Ward, ed. *Sex and Education: A Reply to Dr. E. H. Clarke's "Sex in Education."* Boston: Roberts, 1874.

Howes, Anna G. *Health Statistics of Women College Graduates: Report of a Special Committee of the Association of Collegiate Alumnae.* Boston: Wright and Potter, 1885.

"Illness as Cause of College Failures." *Hygeia* 4 (1926): 413.

Jacobi, Mary Putnam. *The Question of Rest for Women during Menstruation.* New York: Putnam's, 1877.

Keeling, Richard P. "AIDS on the College Campus: Introduction." *Journal of American College Health* 35, no. 3 (1986): 123–26.

Kerns, Harry N. "Cadet Problems." *Mental Hygiene* 7 (1923): 688–93.

Kerns, Harry N. "Management of Acute Mental-Hygiene Problems." *Mental Hygiene* 9 (1925): 273–81.

King, Edith Shatto. "Health Insurance in a Student Community." *Survey* 36 (1916): 619–20.

Kinsey, Alfred C. *Sexual Behavior in the Human Female.* Philadelphia: Saunders, 1953.

Kinsey, Alfred C. *Sexual Behavior in the Human Male.* Philadelphia: Saunders, 1948.

Kodama, Cathy, and Mary O'Donnell. *AIDS Education on the College Campus: A Practical Guide.* Berkeley: Health Promotion Office, University of California, 1987.

Legge, Robert T. "Students' Health Insurance at the University of California." *California State Journal of Medicine* 15, no. 4 (1917): 102–4.

Legge, Robert T. "Students' Health Insurance at the University of California." In *Proceedings of the Conference on Social Insurance, Called by the International Association of Industrial Accident Boards and Commissions*, 505–11, 519–47. Washington, D.C.: U.S. Government Printing Office, 1917.

Long, Esmond R. "The Tuberculosis Experience of the United States Army in World War II." *American Review of Tuberculosis* 55 (1947): 28–37.

Long, Esmond R. "Tuberculosis in College Students, with Special Reference to Tuberculin Testing." *Journal-Lancet*, n.s. 55 (1937): 201–3.

Long, Esmond R., and Florence Seibert. "The Incidence of Tuberculosis Infection in American College Students." *Journal of the American Medical Association* 108 (1937): 1761–65.

MacKeag, Anna J. "Methods in Use in Colleges for Women for the Maintenance and Advancement of the Health of Students." *Woman's Medical Journal* 23 (1913): 199.

McKenzie, R. Tait. *Exercise in Education and Medicine.* Philadelphia: Saunders, 1909.

McKenzie, R. Tait. "Physical Education at the University of Pennsylvania—from 1904 to 1931—and the Gates Plan." *Research Quarterly* 3 (1932): 19–21.

McKenzie, R. Tait. "The Search for Physical Perfection." In *University Lectures Delivered by Members of the Faculty in the Free Public Lecture Course, 1914–1915*, 409–19. Philadelphia: University of Pennsylvania, 1915.

Menninger, Karl A. "Adaptation Difficulties in College Students." *Mental Hygiene* 11 (1927): 519–35.

Meredith, Florence. "The Administration of Mental Hygiene in Colleges." *Mental Hygiene* 11 (1927): 241–52.

Meyers, J. Arthur. "Types of Tuberculosis Lesions Found in the Chests of Students of Nursing and Medicine." *American Review of Tuberculosis* 28 (1933): 93–117.

Meyers, J. Arthur, and L. M. Kernkamp. "Tuberculosis among Boys and Girls in their Teens." *American Review of Tuberculosis* 21 (1930): 509–31.

Miller, Fred N. "Off to College." *Hygeia* 5 (1927): 500–502.

Moore, Norman S., and John Summerskill. *Health Services in American Colleges and Universities, 1953*. Ithaca: Cornell University Press, 1954.

Morris, Earl F. "Going to College for Your Health." *Hygeia* 8 (1930): 801–4.

Mosher, Clelia Duel. "Concerning the Size of Women: Preliminary Note with Special Reference to Height." *California State Journal of Medicine* 19 (1921): 53–54.

Mosher, Clelia Duel. *Health and the Woman Movement*. New York: Young Women's Christian Associations, 1916.

Mosher, Clelia Duel. "The Height of College Women." *Medical Woman's Journal* 28 (1921): 274–76.

Mosher, Clelia Duel. *The Mosher Survey: Sexual Attitudes of Forty-five Victorian Women*. New York: Arno, 1980.

Mosher, Clelia Duel. "The Muscular Strength of College Women." *Journal of the American Medical Association* 70 (1918): 140–42.

Mosher, Clelia Duel. "The Physical Training of Women in Relation to Functional Periodicity." *Woman's Medical Journal* 25, no. 4 (1915): 3–5, 9, 11.

Mosher, Clelia Duel. "A Physiologic Treatment of Congestive Dysmenorrhea and Kindred Disorders Associated with Menstrual Function." *Journal of the American Medical Association* 62 (1914): 1297–1301.

Mosher, Clelia Duel. "The Schematogram—A New Method of Graphically Recording Posture and Changes in the Contours of the Body." *School and Society* 1 (1915): 642–45.

Mosher, Clelia Duel. "Some of the Causal Factors in the Increased Height of College Women." *Journal of the American Medical Association* 81 (1923): 535–38.

Mosher, Clelia Duel. *Woman's Physical Freedom*. New York: Woman's Press, 1923.

Nash, Ethel M. "The College Physician's Role in Sex Education." *Journal of the American College Health Association* 15, supplement (1967): 66–71.

National Student Association. *Gays on Campus*. Washington, D.C.: National Student Association, 1975.

National Tuberculosis Association. *Report of the Committee on Tuberculosis among Negroes*. New York: National Tuberculosis Association, 1937.

National Tuberculosis Association. *Tuberculosis and the 'Teen Age*. New York: National Tuberculosis Association, 1927.

Newcomer, Mabel. "Physical Development of Vassar College Students, 1884–1920." *Publications of the American Statistical Association* 17, no. 136 (1921): 976–82.

Nicholson, Edna. *A Study of Tuberculosis Mortality among Young Women*. New York: National Tuberculosis Association, 1932.

O'Hagan, Annie. "The Athletic Girl." *Munsey's*, August 1901, 729–38.

Palmer, George Herbert, and Alice Freeman Palmer. *The Teacher: Essays and Addresses on Education*. Boston: Houghton Mifflin, 1908.

Paton, Stewart. *Education in War and Peace*. New York: Hoeber, 1920.

Pilpel, Harriet F., and Nancy F. Wechsler. "Birth Control, Teenagers, and the Law." *Family Planning Perspectives* 1, no. 1 (1969): 29–35.

"Plain Facts about Health and Disease." *Hygeia* 6 (1928): 406–7.

President's Commission on Higher Education. *Higher Education for American Democracy*. Vol. 1, *Establishing the Goals*. New York: Harper, 1948.

Proceedings of the First National Conference on Race Betterment. Battle Creek, Mich.: Race Betterment Society, 1914.

Proceedings of the National Conference on College Hygiene. New York: National Tuberculosis Association, 1931.

The Prytaneans: An Oral History of the Prytanean Society and Its Members and Their University, 1901–1920. Berkeley, Calif.: Prytanean Alumnae, 1970.

Raycroft, Joseph E. "Safeguarding the Health of College Students." *Science*, 15 May 1914, 707–11.

Report of the United States Interdepartmental Social Hygiene Board for Fiscal Year Ended June 30, 1920. Washington, D.C.: U.S. Government Printing Office, 1921.

Richardson, Sophia F. "Tendencies in Athletics for Women in Colleges and Universities." *Popular Science Monthly* 50 (1896–97): 517–26.

Rickert, Edith. "Has the College Injured the Health of Girls?" *Ladies' Home Journal*, January1912, 11–12.

Richmond, Winifred. "Mental Hygiene in the Colleges." *Journal of the American Medical Association* 93 (1929): 1936–39.

Riggs, A. F., and W. B. Terhune. "Mental Health of College Women." *Mental Hygiene* 12 (1928): 559–68.

Ritter, Mary Bennett. *More Than Gold in California, 1849–1933*. Berkeley, Calif.: Professional, 1933.

Robinson, Kent E. "The Attack on Student Services." *New Directions for Higher Education* 1, no. 3 (1973): 1–4.

Rorer, S. T. "What College Girls Eat." *Ladies' Home Journal*, November 1905, 13–14.

Rudolph, Frederick. *The American College and University: A History*. New York: Knopf, 1962.

Ruggles, Arthur Hiler. *Mental Health: Past, Present, and Future*. Providence, R.I.: Williams and Wilkins, 1934.

Ryan, Calvin T. "If I Were Selecting a College." *Hygeia* 12 (1934): 778–80.

Ryan, Marie B. "A College Training in Health." *Hygeia* 4 (1926): 575–78.

Rydell, Robert W. *All the World's a Fair: Visions of Empire at American International Expositions, 1876–1916*. Chicago: University of Chicago Press, 1984.

Sargent, Dudley Allen. "The Physical Development of Women." *Scribner's*, February 1889, 172–85.

Sargent, Dudley Allen. "The Relation of Physical Education to Race Betterment." In *Proceedings of the First National Conference on Race Betterment*, 104–6. Battle Creek, Mich.: Gage, 1914.

Sargent, Dudley Allen. *Dudley Allen Sargent: An Autobiography*. Ed. Ledyard W. Sargent. Philadelphia: Lea and Febiger, 1927.

Sarrel, Philip M., and Lorna J. Sarrel. "Birth Control Services and Sex Counseling at Yale." *Family Planning Perspectives* 3, no. 3 (1971): 33–36.

Schoenfeld, Eugene. *Doctor Hip Pocrates: Advice Your Family Doctor Never Gave You*. New York: Grove, 1969.

Shaw, Albert. "Physical Culture at Wellesley." *American Review of Reviews* 6 (1892): 545–49.

Shepard, Charles E. "Campaign against Tuberculosis in College Students." *American Journal of Public Health* 25, no. 10 (1935): 1118–24.

Slosson, Edwin E. *Great American Universities.* New York: Macmillan, 1910.

Smiley, D. F. "The Health of Your Boy in College." *Hygeia* 4 (1926): 554–58.

Smith, David E. "Runaways and Their Health Problems in Haight-Ashbury during the Summer of 1967." *American Journal of Public Health* 59, no. 11 (1969): 2046–50.

Smith, Mary Roberts. "Statistics of College and Non-College Women." *Publications of the American Statistical Association* 7 (1900–1901): 1–26.

Snow, Glenadine. "Health Problems of Women Students." *Proceedings of the Fifth Annual Meeting of the American Student Health Association,* 1925, 8–11.

Soper, George A. "The Epidemic of Typhoid Fever at Ithaca, N.Y." *Journal of the New England Water Works Association* 18, no. 4 (1905): 431–61.

Soule, Annah May. "Relation of the School and College to Health." *School Review* 11 (1903): 817–26.

Storey, Thomas A. "The Colleges Look at Hygiene." *Journal of Social Hygiene* 17, no. 7 (1931): 381–92.

Storey, Thomas A. *The Status of Hygiene Programs in Institutions of Higher Education in the United States.* Stanford, Calif.: Stanford University Press, 1927.

Storey, Thomas A. "A Summary of the United States Interdepartmental Social Hygiene Board." *Social Hygiene* 7, no. 1 (1921): 59–76.

Storey, Thomas A. "The Work of the United States Interdepartmental Social Hygiene Board." *Social Hygiene* 5, no. 4 (1919): 441–60.

Storey, Thomas A., Frederic Allen Wolf, and Julian Park, eds. *Fourth International Congress on School Hygiene.* Buffalo, N.Y.: Courier, 1914.

Straus, Robert, and Selden Bacon. *Drinking in College.* New Haven: Yale University Press, 1953.

Studley, Mary J. *What Our Girls Ought to Know.* New York: Holbrook, 1878.

Sundwall, John. "The Interrelationship between Physical Education and Students' Health Service." *American Physical Education Review,* 1921, 172–79.

Sundwall, John. "The Teaching of College Hygiene." *American Journal of Public Health* 17, no. 1 (1927): 48–57.

Sundwall, John. "What Physical Education Should Contribute to Race Betterment." In *Proceedings of the Third Race Betterment Conference,* 704–14. Battle Creek, Mich.: Race Betterment Foundation, 1928.

Szasz, Thomas S. "College Psychiatry: A Critique." *Comprehensive Psychiatry* 9, no. 1 (1968): 81–88.

Szasz, Thomas S. "The Psychiatrist as Double Agent." *Trans-Action* 4 (1967): 18–24.

Thomas, M. Carey. "Present Tendencies in Women's College and University Education." *Educational Review* 35 (1908): 64–85.

Thompson, C. Mildred. "The Value of Mental Hygiene in the College." *Mental Hygiene* 11 (1927): 225–40.

Thurston, Linda. *Birth Control, Abortion, and Venereal Disease.* Cambridge, Mass.: Resist, 1970.

Trussell, James, and Steve Chandler. *The Loving Book.* Charlotte, N.C.: Red Clay, 1971.

Turner, H. Spencer. "New Realities: The Challenge to Change." *Journal of the American College Health Association* 30, no. 1 (1981):7–9.

University of Pennsylvania. *The Dormitory System as Designed by Cope and Stewardson, Architects.* Philadelphia: privately printed, 1895.

Wedge, Bryan M., ed. *Psychosocial Problems of College Men.* New Haven: Yale University Press, 1958.

Wood, Thomas D. "How Much Do College Graduates Know about Health?" *Hygeia* 2 (1924): 113–14.

SECONDARY SOURCES

Abt, Henry Edward. *Ithaca.* Ithaca, N.Y.: Kellogg, 1926.

Allmendinger, David F., Jr. "The Dangers of Antebellum Student Life." *Journal of Social History* 7, no. 1 (1973): 75–85.

Allmendinger, David F., Jr. *Paupers and Scholars: The Transformation of Student Life in Nineteenth-Century New England.* New York: St. Martin's, 1975.

Anderson, Eric, and Alfred A. Moss Jr. *Dangerous Donations: Northern Philanthropy and Southern Black Education, 1902–1930.* Columbia: University of Missouri Press, 1999.

Angelo, Richard. "The Students at the University of Pennsylvania and the Temple College of Philadelphia, 1873–1906: Some Notes on Schooling, Class, and Social Mobility in the Late Nineteenth Century." *History of Education Quarterly* 19, no. 2 (1979): 179–205.

Appel, Toby. "Physiology in American Women's Colleges: The Rise and Decline of a Female Subculture." *Isis* 85, no. 1 (1994): 26–56.

Bailey, Beth. *From Front Porch to Back Seat: Courtship in Twentieth-Century America.* Baltimore: Johns Hopkins University Press, 1988.

Bailey, Beth. *Sex in the Heartland.* Cambridge: Harvard University Press, 1999.

Baltzell, E. Digby. *Philadelphia Gentlemen: The Making of a National Upper Class.* New Brunswick, N.J.: Transaction, 1989.

Barker-Benfield, Ben. "The Spermatic Economy: A Nineteenth-Century View of Sexuality." *Feminist Studies* 1, no. 1 (1972): 45–74.

Bates, Barbara. *Bargaining for Life: A Social History of Tuberculosis, 1876–1938.* Philadelphia: University of Pennsylvania Press, 1992.

Beardsley, Edward H. *A History of Neglect: Health Care for Blacks and Mill Workers in the Twentieth-Century South.* Knoxville: University of Tennessee Press, 1987.

Bederman, Gail. *Manliness and Civilization: A Cultural History of Gender and Race in the United States, 1880–1917.* Chicago: University of Chicago Press, 1995.

Berry, Romeyn. *Behind the Ivy: Fifty Years in One University with Visits to Sundry Others.* Ithaca: Cornell University Press, 1950.

Bishop, Morris. *A History of Cornell.* Ithaca: Cornell University Press, 1962.

Bittel, Carla Jean. "The Science of Women's Rights: The Medical and Political Worlds of Mary Putnam Jacobi." Ph.D. diss., Cornell University, 2003.

The Black Women Oral History Project. Cambridge, Mass.: Schlesinger Library, Radcliffe College, 1984.

Boynton, Ruth. "The First Fifty Years: A History of the American College Health Association." *Journal of the American College Health Association* 19, no. 5 (1971): 269–285.

Boynton, Ruth. "Historical Development of College Health Services." *Student Medicine* 10 (1962): 294–305.

Brandt, Allan. *No Magic Bullet: A Social History of Venereal Disease in the United States since 1880.* New York: Oxford University Press, 1985.

Bristow, Nancy. *Making Men Moral: Social Engineering during the Great War.* New York: New York University Press, 1996.

Brumberg, Joan Jacobs. *The Body Project: An Intimate History of American Girls.* New York: Vintage, 1998.

Brumberg, Joan Jacobs. *Mission for Life.* New York: Free Press, 1980.

Bullough, Vern. *Science in the Bedroom: A History of Sex Research.* New York: Basic Books, 1994.

Burbick, Joan. *Healing the Republic: The Language of Health and the Culture of Nationalism in Nineteenth-Century America.* New York: Cambridge University Press, 1994.

Caron, Simone M. "Birth Control and the Black Community in the 1960s: Genocide or Power Politics?" *Journal of Social History* 31, no. 3 (1998): 545–59.

Cheyney, Edward Potts. *History of the University of Pennsylvania, 1740–1940.* Philadelphia: University of Pennsylvania Press, 1940.

Christmas, William A. "The Evolution of Medical Services for Students at Colleges and Universities in the United States." *Journal of American College Health* 43, no. 6 (1995): 241–46.

Christmas, William A., and John M. Dorman. "The Storey of College Health Hygiene: Thomas A. Storey (1875–1943) and the Promotion of Hygiene." *Journal of American College Health* 45, no. 1 (1996): 27–35.

Clifford, Geraldine Jonçich, ed. *Lone Voyagers: Academic Women in Coeducational Universities, 1870–1937.* New York: Feminist, 1989.

Cline, David. *Creating Choice: A Community Responds to the Need for Abortion and Birth Control, 1961–1973.* New York: Palgrave, 2006.

Cohen, Patricia Cline. *The Murder of Helen Jewett.* New York: Vintage, 1998.

Cohen, Sol. "The Mental Hygiene Movement and the Development of Personality: Changing Conceptions of the American College and University, 1920–1940." *History of Higher Education Annual* 2 (1982): 65–101.

Conable, Charlotte. *Women at Cornell: The Myth of Equal Education.* Ithaca: Cornell University Press, 1977.

Cravens, Hamilton. *The Triumph of Evolution: American Scientists and the Heredity-Environment Controversy, 1900–1941.* Philadelphia: University of Pennsylvania Press, 1978.

Dain, Norman. *Clifford W. Beers: Advocate for the Insane.* Pittsburgh: University of Pittsburgh Press, 1980.

Darby, Robert. "The Masturbation Taboo and the Rise of Routine Male Circumcision: A Review of the Historiography." *Journal of Social History* 36, no. 3 (2003): 737–57.

Deluzio, Crista Jean. "'New Girls for Old': Female Adolescence in American Scientific Thought, 1870–1930." Ph.D. diss., Brown University, 1999.

Deutsch, Albert. *The Story of GAP.* New York: Group for the Advancement of Psychiatry, 1959.

Digginbotham, Ian Robert. *Keeping America Sane: Psychiatry and Eugenics in the United States and Canada, 1880–1940.* Ithaca: Cornell University Press, 1997.

Diggs, Marylynne. "Romantic Friends or a 'Different Race of Creatures'? The Representation of Lesbian Pathology in Nineteenth Century America." *Feminist Studies* 21, no. 2 (1995): 317–40.

Dilley, James W. "Development of the Structure of the American College Health Association." *Journal of the American College Health Association* 28, no. 6 (1971): 354–58.

Dilley, Patrick. *Gay Man on Campus: A History of Non-Heterosexual College Men, 1945–2000.* New York: Routledge Falmer, 2002.

Drewry, Henry N. *Stand and Prosper: Black Colleges and Their Students.* Princeton: Princeton University Press, 2001.

Duffy, John. "Mental Strain and Overpressure in the Schools: A Nineteenth-Century Viewpoint." *Journal of the History of Medicine and Allied Sciences* 23, no. 1 (1968): 63–79.

Duke, Alex. *Importing Oxbridge: English Residential Colleges and American Universities.* New Haven: Yale University Press, 1996.

Elliott, Orrin Leslie. *Stanford University: The First Twenty-five Years.* Stanford, Calif.: Stanford University Press, 1937.

Engel, J. W. "Early Psychiatry at Yale: Milton C. Winternitz and the Founding of the Department of Psychiatry and Mental Hygiene." *Yale Journal of Biology and Medicine* 67, nos. 1–2 (1994): 33–47.

Engel, Jonathan. *Doctors and Reformers: Discussion and Debate over Health Policy, 1925–1950.* Columbia: University of South Carolina Press, 2002.

Engelhardt, Tristam H. "The Disease of Masturbation: Values and the Concept of Disease." *Bulletin of the History of Medicine* 48, no. 2 (1974): 234–38.

English, Daylanne K. *Unnatural Selections: Eugenics in American Modernism and the Harlem Renaissance.* Chapel Hill: University of North Carolina Press, 2004.

Ettling, John. *The Germ of Laziness: Rockefeller Philanthropy and Public Health in the New South.* Cambridge: Harvard University Press, 1981.

Fairchild, Amy. *Science at the Borders: Immigrant Medical Inspection and the Shaping of the Modern Industrial Labor Force.* Baltimore: Johns Hopkins University Press, 2003.

Falk, I. S. "Medical Care in the USA—1932–1972." *Milbank Memorial Fund Quarterly* 51, no. 11 (1973): 1–39.

Faraghar, John Mack, and Florence Howe, eds. *Women and Higher Education in American History: Essays from the Mount Holyoke College Sesquicentennial Symposia.* New York: Norton, 1988.

Fass, Paula S. *The Damned and the Beautiful: American Youth in the 1920s.* New York: Basic Books, 1977.

Fass, Paula S. "Making and Remaking an Event: The Leopold and Loeb Case in American Culture." *Journal of American History* 80, no. 3 (1993): 919–51.

Fass, Paula S. *Outside In: Minorities and the Transformation of American Education.* New York: Oxford University Press, 1989.

Feldberg, Georgina D. *Disease and Class: Tuberculosis and the Shaping of North American Society.* New Brunswick, N.J.: Rutgers University Press, 1995.

Fletcher, Robert Samuel. *A History of Oberlin College from Its Foundation through the Civil War.* Oberlin, Ohio: Oberlin College, 1943.

Franklin, Paul B. "Jew Boys, Queer Boys: Rhetorics of Antisemitism and Homophobia in the Trial of Nathan 'Babe' Leopold, Jr. and Richard 'Dickie' Loeb." In *Queer Theory and the Jewish Question*, ed. Daniel Boyarin, Daniel Itzkovitz, and Ann Pellegrini, 121–48. New York: Columbia University Press, 2003.

Friedman, Lawrence J. *Menninger: The Family and the Clinic.* Lawrence: University Press of Kansas, 1990.

Fuess, Claude Moore. *Amherst: The Story of a New England College.* Boston: Little, Brown, 1935.

Garrow, David J. *Liberty and Sexuality: The Right to Privacy and the Making of* Roe v. Wade. Berkeley: University of California Press, 1998.

Gordon, Colin. *Dead on Arrival: The Politics of Health Care in Twentieth-Century America.* Princeton: Princeton University Press, 2003.

Gordon, Lynn D. *Gender and Higher Education in the Progressive Era.* New Haven: Yale University Press, 1990.

Grant, Julia. "A 'Real Boy' and Not a Sissy: Gender, Childhood, and Masculinity, 1890–1940." *Journal of Social History* 37, no. 4 (2004): 829–51.

Green, Harvey. *Fit for America: Health, Fitness, Sport, and American Society.* New York: Pantheon, 1986.

Grob, Gerald. *Mental Illness and American Society, 1875–1940.* Princeton: Princeton University Press, 1983.

Gunn, Jennifer L. "Factory Work for Doctors: The Early Years of the Section on Industrial Medicine and Public Health of the College of Physicians of Philadelphia." *Transactions and Studies of the College of Physicians of Philadelphia* 17 (1995): 61–93.

Gustav-Wrathall, John Donald. *Take the Young Stranger by the Hand: Same-Sex Relations and the YWCA.* Chicago: University of Chicago Press, 1998.

Haller, John S., and Robin M. Haller, *The Physician and Sexuality in Victorian America.* New York: Norton, 1974.

Harris, Dorothy. *History of Ithaca's Water and Sewer Systems.* Ithaca, N.Y.: Department of Public Works, Water and Sewer Division, 1956.

Hendricks, Rickey. *A Model for National Health Care: The History of Kaiser Permanente.* New Brunswick, N.J.: Rutgers University Press, 1993.

Herbst, Jurgen. *And Sadly Teach: Teacher Education and Professionalization in American Culture.* Madison: University of Wisconsin Press, 1989.

Herman, Debra. "College and After: The Vassar Experiment in Women's Education, 1861–1924." Ph.D. diss., Stanford University, 1979.

Hoffman, Beatrix. *The Wages of Sickness: The Politics of Health Insurance in Progressive America.* Chapel Hill: University of North Carolina Press, 2001.

Hofstader, Richard. *The Age of Reform.* New York: Knopf, 1955.

Holt, Marilyn. *Linoleum, Better Babies, and the Modern Farm Woman, 1890–1930.* Albuquerque: University of New Mexico Press, 1995.

Horowitz, Helen Lefkowitz. *Alma Mater: Design and Experience in the Women's Colleges from Their Beginnings to the 1930s.* Boston: Beacon, 1984.

Horowitz, Helen Lefkowitz. *Campus Life: Undergraduate Cultures from the End of the Eighteenth Century to the Present.* Chicago: University of Chicago Press, 1987.

Johnson, John W. Griswold v. Connecticut: *Birth Control and the Constitutional Right of Privacy.* Lawrence: University Press of Kansas, 2005.

Jones, James H. *Bad Blood: The Tuskegee Syphilis Experiment—A Tragedy of Race and Medicine.* New York: Free Press, 1981.

Jones, Kathleen W. *Taming the Troublesome Child: American Families, Child Guidance, and the Limits of Psychiatric Authority.* Cambridge: Harvard University Press, 1999.

Kammen, Carol. *The Peopling of Tompkins County: A Social History.* Interlaken, N.Y.: Heart of the Lakes, 1985.

Karabel, Jerome. *The Chosen: The Hidden History of Admission and Exclusion at Harvard, Yale, and Princeton.* New York: Houghton Mifflin, 2005.

Kazan, John F. *Houdini, Tarzan, and the Perfect Man: The White Male Body and the Challenge of Modernity in America.* New York: Hill and Wang, 2001.

Keeling, Richard P. "College Health Responds to HIV: Hard Lessons and a Rich Heritage." *Journal of American College Health* 43, no. 6 (1995): 271–72.

Kerber, Linda. *Women of the Republic: Intellect and Ideology in Revolutionary America.* Chapel Hill: University of North Carolina Press, 1986.

Kett, Joseph. *Rites of Passage: Adolescence in America, 1790 to the Present.* New York: Basic Books, 1977.

Kevles, Daniel. *In the Name of Eugenics: Genetics and the Uses of Human Heredity.* New York: Knopf, 1985.

Kimmelman, Barbara A. "The American Breeders' Association: Genetics and Eugenics in an Agricultural Context, 1903–13." *Social Studies of Science* 13, no. 2 (1983): 163–204.

Kline, Wendy. *Building a Better Race: Gender, Sexuality, and Eugenics from the Turn of the Century to the Baby Boom.* Berkeley: University of California Press, 2001.

Ladd, Tony, and James A. Mathisen. *Muscular Christianity: Evangelical Protestants and the Development of American Sport.* Grand Rapids, Mich.: Baker, 1999.

Larson, Edward J. *Sex, Race, and Science: Eugenics in the Deep South.* Baltimore: Johns Hopkins University Press, 1996.

Lasser, Carol, ed.. *Educating Men and Women Together: Coeducation in a Changing World.* Urbana: University of Illinois Press, 1987.

Leach, William. *True Love and Perfect Union: The Feminist Reform of Sex and Science.* New York: Basic Books, 1980.

Leavitt, Judith Walzer. *Typhoid Mary: Captive to the Public Health.* Boston: Beacon, 1996.

Lemann, Nicolas. *The Big Test: The Secret History of American Meritocracy.* New York: Farrar, Straus, and Giroux, 1999.

Lerner, Barron H. "Constructing Medical Indications: The Sterilization of Women with Heart Disease or Tuberculosis, 1905–1935." *Journal of the History of Medicine and Allied Sciences* 49, no. 3 (1994): 362–79.

Lerner, Barron H. *Contagion and Confinement: Controlling Tuberculosis along the Skid Road.* Baltimore: Johns Hopkins University Press, 1998.

Levine, David O. *The American College and the Culture of Aspiration, 1915–1940.* Ithaca: Cornell University Press, 1986.

Levine, Murray, and Julius Wishner. "The Case Records of the Psychological Clinic at the University of Pennsylvania." *Journal of the History of the Behavioral Sciences* 13, no. 1 (1977): 59–66.

Lord, Alexandra M. "Models of Masculinity: Sex Education, the United States Public Health Service, and the YMCA, 1919–1924." *Journal of the History of Medicine and Allied Sciences* 58, no. 2 (2003): 123–52.

Lord, Alexandra M. "Naturally Clean and Wholesome: Women, Sex Education, and the United States Public Health Service, 1918–1928." *Social History of Medicine* 17, no. 3 (2004): 423–41.

Lowe, Margaret A. *Looking Good: College Women and Body Image, 1875–1930.* Baltimore: Johns Hopkins University Press, 2003.

Lunbeck, Elizabeth. *The Psychiatric Persuasion: Knowledge, Gender, and Power in Modern America.* Princeton: Princeton University Press, 1994.

Marcus, Alan I. "The South's Native Foreigners: Hookworm as a Factor in Southern Distinctiveness." In *Disease and Distinctiveness in the American South,* ed. Todd L. Savitt and James Harvey Young, 79–99. Knoxville: University of Tennessee Press, 1988.

Marmor, Theodore R. "The Politics of Universal Health Insurance: Lessons from the Past?" *Journal of Interdisciplinary History* 26, no. 4 (1996): 671–79.

McCarthy, Michael P. *Typhoid and the Politics of Public Health in Nineteenth-Century Philadelphia.* Philadelphia: American Philosophical Society, 1987.

McGuigan, Dorothy Gies. *A Dangerous Experiment: 100 Years of Women at the University of Michigan.* Ann Arbor: University of Michigan, 1970.

Meckel, Richard A. "Going to School, Getting Sick: The Social and Medical Construction of School Diseases in the Late Nineteenth Century." In *Formative Years: Children's Health in the United States, 1880–2000,* ed. Alexandra Minna Stern and Howard Markel, 185–207. Ann Arbor: University of Michigan Press, 2002.

Meier, August, and Elliott Rudwick. *Black History and the Historical Profession.* Urbana: University of Illinois Press, 1986.

Meyerson, Martin, and Dilys Pegler Winegrad. *Gladly Learn and Gladly Teach: Franklin and His Heirs at the University of Pennsylvania, 1740–1976.* Philadelphia: University of Pennsylvania Press, 1978.

Mitchell, Michelle. *Righteous Propagation: African Americans and the Politics of Racial Destiny after Reconstruction.* Chapel Hill: University of North Carolina Press, 2004.

Montgomery, Rebecca S. *The Politics of Education in the New South: Women and Reform in Georgia.* Baton Rouge: Louisiana State University Press, 2006.

Moran, Jeffrey P. *Teaching Sex: The Shaping of Adolescence in the Twentieth Century.* Cambridge: Harvard University Press, 2000.

Morantz-Sanchez, Regina Markell. *Sympathy and Science: Women Physicians in American Medicine.* New York: Oxford University Press, 1985.

More, Ellen Singer. *Restoring the Balance: Women Physicians and the Profession of Medicine.* Cambridge: Harvard University Press, 1999.

Morgen, Sandra. *Into Our Own Hands: The Women's Health Movement in the United States, 1969–1990.* New Brunswick, N.J.: Rutgers University Press, 2001.

Muncy, Robyn. *Creating a Female Dominion in American Reform, 1890–1935.* New York: Oxford University Press, 1991.

Myers, J. Arthur. *Masters of Medicine: An Historical Sketch of the College of Medical Sciences, University of Minnesota, 1888–1966.* St. Louis: Green, 1968.

Neuman, R. P. "Masturbation, Madness, and the Modern Concepts of Childhood and Adolescence." *Journal of Social History* 8, no. 3 (1976): 1–27.

Nidiffer, Jana. *Pioneering Deans of Women: More Than Wise and Pious Matrons.* New York: Teachers College Press, 2000.

Nissenbaum, Stephen. *Sex, Diet, and Debility in Jacksonian America.* Westport, Conn.: Greenwood, 1980.

Numbers, Ronald L. *Almost Persuaded: American Physicians and Compulsory Health Insurance, 1912–1920.* Baltimore: Johns Hopkins University Press, 1978.

Nugent, Angela. "Fit for Work: The Introduction of Physical Examinations in Industry." *Bulletin of the History of Medicine* 57, no. 4 (1983): 578–95.

Ott, Katherine. *Fevered Lives: Tuberculosis in American Culture since 1870.* Cambridge: Harvard University Press, 1996.

Owens, Larry. "Pure and Sound Government: Laboratories, Playing Fields, and Gymnasia in the Nineteenth-Century Search for Order." *Isis* 76, no. 2 (1985):182–94.

Park, Roberta. "Physiologists, Physicians, and Physical Educators: Nineteenth Century Biology and Exercise, *Hygienic* and *Educative.*" *Journal of Sport History* 14, no. 1 (1987): 28–60.

Park, Roberta. "Research Note: Edward M. Hartwell and Physical Training at the Johns Hopkins University, 1879–1890." *Journal of Sport History* 14, no. 1 (1987): 108–19.

Parsons, Gail Pat. "Equal Treatment for All: American Medical Remedies for Male Sexual Problems, 1850–1900." *Journal of the History of Medicine and Allied Sciences* 32, no. 1 (1977): 55–71.

Patrick, Kevin. "The History and Current Status of College Health." In *Principles and Practice of Student Health*, vol. 3, *College Health*, ed. Helen M. Wallace et al. Oakland, Calif.: Third Party, 1992.

Paul, Diane. *Controlling Human Heredity: 1865 to the Present.* Atlantic Highlands, N.J.: Humanities, 1995.

Pernick, Martin. *The Black Stork: Eugenics and the Death of "Defective" Babies in American Medicine and Motion Pictures since 1915.* New York: Oxford University Press, 1996.

Pols, Johannes Coenraad. "Managing the Mind: The Culture of American Mental Hygiene, 1910–1950." Ph.D. diss., University of Pennsylvania, 1997.

Prescott, Heather Munro. *"A Doctor of Their Own": The History of Adolescent Medicine.* Cambridge: Harvard University Press, 1998.

Pressman, Jack. *Last Resort: Psychosurgery and the Limits of Medicine.* Cambridge: Cambridge University Press, 1998.

Raycroft, Joseph E. "History and Development of Student Health Programs in Colleges and Universities." *Proceedings of the Twenty-first Annual Meeting of the American Student Health Association*, 1940, 37–43.

Robinson, Harry G., and Hazel Ruth Edwards. *The Long Walk: The Placemaking Legacy of Howard University.* Washington, D.C.: Moorland-Spingarn Research Center, Howard University, 1996.

Roemer, Milton I. "I. S. Falk, the Committee on the Costs of Medical Care, and the Drive for National Health Insurance." *American Journal of Public Health* 75, no. 8 (1985): 841–48.

Rogers, Naomi. "'Caution: The AMA May Be Dangerous to Your Health': The Student Health Organizations (SHO) and American Medicine, 1965–1970." *Radical History Review* 80 (2001): 5–34.

Rorabaugh, W. J. *Berkeley at War: The 1960s.* New York: Oxford University Press, 1989.

Rosen, George. "Contract or Lodge Practice and Its Influence on Medical Attitudes to Health Insurance." *American Journal of Public Health* 67, no. 4 (1977): 374–78.

Rosenberg, Charles E. *The Care of Strangers: The Rise of America's Hospital System.* New York: Basic Books, 1987.

Rosenberg, Charles E. "Sexuality, Class, and Role in Nineteenth-Century America." *American Quarterly* 25, no. 2 (1973): 131–53.

Rosenberg, Rosalind. *Beyond Separate Spheres: Intellectual Roots of Modern Feminism.* New Haven: Yale University Press, 1982

Rosencrantz, Barbara Gutman. *Public Health and the State: Changing Views in Massachusetts.* Cambridge: Harvard University Press, 1972.

Ross, Dorothy. *G. Stanley Hall: The Psychologist as Prophet.* Chicago: University of Chicago Press, 1972.

Rossi, A. M. "Some Pre–World War II Antecedents of Community Mental Health Theory and Practice." *Mental Hygiene* 46 (1962): 78–98.

Rothman, Sheila. *Living in the Shadow of Death: Tuberculosis and the Social Experience of Illness in American History.* New York: Basic Books, 1994.

Rothman, Sheila. *Woman's Proper Place: A History of Changing Practices, 1870 to the Present.* New York: Basic Books, 1978.

Rupke, Nicolaas A. *Richard Owen: Victorian Naturalist.* New Haven: Yale University Press, 1994.

Russett, Cynthia Eagle. *Sexual Science: The Victorian Construction of Womanhood.* Cambridge: Harvard University Press, 1989.

Schoen, Johanna. *Choice and Coercion: Birth Control, Sterilization, and Abortion in Public Health and Welfare.* Chapel Hill: University of North Carolina Press, 2005.

Selden, Steven. "Education Policy and Biological Science: Genetics, Eugenics, and the College Textbook, c. 1908–1931." *Teachers College Record* 87, no. 1 (1985): 35–51.

Sellers, Christopher. *Hazards of the Job: From Industrial Disease to Environmental Health Science.* Chapel Hill: University of North Carolina Press, 1997.

Sethna, Christabelle. "The Evolution of the *Birth Control Handbook:* From Student Peer Education Manual to Feminist Self-Help Text, 1968–1975." *Canadian Bulletin of Medical History* 23, no. 1 (2006): 89–117.

Sethna, Christabelle. "The University of Toronto Health Service, Oral Contraception, and Student Demand for Birth Control, 1960–1970." *Historical Studies in Education* 17, no. 2 (2005): 265–92.

Setran, David P. "Student Religious Life in the 'Era of Secularization': The Intercollegiate YMCA, 1877–1940." *History of Higher Education Annual* 21 (2001): 7–45.

Seymour, Richard B., and David E. Smith. *The Haight-Ashbury Free Medical Clinics: Still Free after All These Years, 1967–1987.* San Francisco: Partisan, 1986.

Shryock, Richard Harrison. *National Tuberculosis Association, 1904–1954: A Study of the Voluntary Health Movement in the United States.* New York: Arno, 1977.

Sicherman, Barbara. "The Paradox of Prudence: Mental Health in the Gilded Age." *Journal of American History* 62, no. 4 (1976): 890–912.

Sicherman, Barbara. *The Quest for Mental Health in America, 1880–1917.* New York: Arno, 1980.

Simmons, Christina. "African Americans and Sexual Victorianism in the Social Hygiene Movement, 1910–1940." *Journal of the History of Sexuality* 4 (1993): 51–75.

Sisler, Carol U., Margaret Hobbie, and Jane Marsh Dieckmann, eds. *Ithaca's Neighborhoods: The Rhine, the Hill, and the Goose Pasture.* Ithaca, N.Y.: Dewitt Historical Society of Tompkins County, 1988.

Smith, David E. *Love Needs Care: A History of San Francisco's Haight-Ashbury Free Medical Clinic.* Boston: Little, Brown, 1971.

Smith, Susan L. *Sick and Tired of Being Sick and Tired: Black Women's Health Activism in America, 1890–1950.* Philadelphia: University of Pennsylvania Press, 1995.

Smith-Rosenberg, Carroll. *Disorderly Conduct: Visions of Gender in Victorian America.* New York: Knopf, 1985.

Solomon, Barbara Miller. *In the Company of Educated Women: A History of Women in Higher Education.* New Haven: Yale University Press, 1985.

Spurlock, John C. "From Reassurance to Irrelevance: Adolescent Psychology and Homosexuality in America." *History of Psychology* 5, no. 1 (2002): 38–51.

Starr, Paul. *The Social Transformation of American Medicine.* New York: Basic Books, 1982.

Stern, Alexandra Minna. *Eugenic Nation: Faults and Frontiers of Better Breeding in Modern America.* Berkeley: University of California Press, 2005.

Stevens, Rosemary. *In Sickness and in Wealth: American Hospitals in the Twentieth Century.* Baltimore: Johns Hopkins University Press, 1989.

Summers, Martin. *Manliness and Its Discontents: The Black Middle Class and the Transformation of Masculinity, 1900–1930.* Chapel Hill: University of North Carolina Press, 2004.

Swanson, Theodor. *The Story of Dick's House.* Lunenburg, Vt.: Stinehour, 1977.

Terry, Jennifer, and Jacqueline Urla, eds., *Deviant Bodies: Critical Perspectives on Difference in Science and Popular Culture.* Bloomington: Indiana University Press, 1995.

Tomes, Nancy. *The Gospel of Germs: Men, Women, and the Microbe in American Life.* Cambridge: Harvard University Press, 1998.

Tracy, Sarah W. *Alcoholism in America: From Reconstruction to Prohibition.* Baltimore: Johns Hopkins University Press, 2004.

Turner, H. Spencer, and Janet L. Hurley, eds. *History and Practice of College Health.* Lexington: University Press of Kentucky, 2002.

Vandenberg-Daves, Jodi. "The Manly Pursuit of a Partnership between the Sexes: The Debate over YMCA Programs for Women and Girls, 1914–1933." *Journal of American History* 78, no. 4 (1992): 1324–46.

Verbrugge, Martha. *Able-Bodied Womanhood: Personal Health and Social Change in Nineteenth-Century Boston.* New York: Oxford University Press, 1988.

Veysey, Laurence R. *The Emergence of the American University.* Chicago: University of Chicago Press, 1965.

Walker, Forrest A. "Americanism versus Sovietism: A Study of the Reaction to the Committee on the Costs of Medical Care." *Bulletin of the History of Medicine* 53, no. 4 (1979): 489–504.

Ward, Thomas J. *Black Physicians in the Jim Crow South.* Fayetteville: University of Arkansas Press, 2003.

Warner, John Harley. "Ideals of Science and Their Discontents in Late Nineteenth-Century American Medicine." *Isis* 82, no. 313 (1991): 454–78.

Welch, J. Edmund. "Pioneering in Health Education and Services at Amherst College." *Journal of the American College Health Association* 30, no. 6 (1982): 289–95.

Whorton, James C. "'Athlete's Heart': The Medical Debate over Athleticism." *Journal of Sport History* 9, no. 1 (1982): 30–52.

Whorton, James C. *Crusaders for Fitness: The History of American Health Reformers.* Princeton: Princeton University Press, 1982.

Wiebe, Robert H. *The Search for Order, 1877–1920.* New York: Hill and Wang, 1967.

Wolters, Raymond. *The New Negro on Campus: Black College Rebellions of the 1920s.* Princeton: Princeton University Press, 1975.

Woody, Thomas. *A History of Women's Education in the United States.* New York: Science, 1929.

Young, James Allen. "Height, Weight, and Health: Anthropometric Study of Human Growth in Nineteenth-Century American Medicine." *Bulletin of the History of Medicine* 53, no. 2 (1979): 214–43.

Zenderland, Leila. *Measuring Minds: Henry Herbert Goddard and the Origins of American Intelligence Tests.* New York: Cambridge University Press, 1998.

Zimmerman, Jonathan. "'One's Total World View Comes into Play': America's Culture War over Alcohol Education, 1945–1964." *History of Education Quarterly* 42, no. 4 (2002): 471–92.

Zschoche, Sue. "Dr. Clarke Revisited: Science, True Womanhood, and Female Collegiate Education." *History of Education Quarterly* 29, no. 4 (1989): 545–69.

Index